REIKI FOR SPIRITUAL HEALING

REIKI

FOR

SPIRITUAL

HEALING

BRETT BEVELL

CROSSING PRESS
BERKELEY

Published in the United States by Crossing Press, an imprint of the Crown Publishing Group,
a division of Random House, Inc., New York.
www.crownpublishing.com
www.tenspeed.com

Crossing Press and the Crossing Press colophon are registered trademarks of Random House, Inc.

Elder Futhark font by Curtis Clark.

Library of Congress Cataloging-in-Publication Data
Bevell, Brett.
Reiki for spiritual healing / by Brett Bevell.
    p. cm.
Summary: "A guide to focusing the energy of Reiki—traditionally used for healing the body—
toward healing the spirit, from Reiki master Brett Bevell"—Provided by publisher.
  Includes bibliographical references and index.
1. Spiritual healing. 2. Reiki (Healing system) I. Title.
  BL65.M4B44 2009
  131—dc22
                                        2009010741
ISBN 978-1-58091-194-8

Cover design by theBookDesigners
Text design by Michael Cutter

First Edition

146119709

*To Helema Kadir and all the beauty she has brought into my life.
And to the spirit of Mikao Usui for bringing
to humanity the wonderful gift of Reiki.*

Contents

Acknowledgments

I owe my deepest gratitude to the spirit of Mikao Usui, Reiki's founder, for bringing the gift of Reiki to this planet and also for overseeing its continued evolution into more advanced forms through the teachings he has offered me. I also wish to humbly thank the archangel Raphael for assisting in this process. My deep thanks go out as well to my dear Reiki Master and shaman friends Carolion, James Philip, Michele Denis, Kathy Fitzgerald, Noelle Adamo, and Hethyrre for their continued support and advice.

I extend sincere thanks to Jo Ann Deck, Lisa Westmoreland, and Brie Mazurek at Crossing Press for their belief in my work and their continued support.

I owe many thanks to Lois Guarino at Omega Institute for supporting me in teaching classes to the Omega staff; to Andy Milford for his constant Web assistance; to the entire Omega Institute Programming Department for having confidence in me as an Omega Institute workshop instructor; and to Donia Foster for supporting my Reiki group healing classes in the Omega Rest and Rejuvenation Retreats program, where much of the information in this book was put to use.

And, of course, I wish to thank the love of my life, Helema Kadir, for keeping me grounded through all of this.

Introduction

I wrote this book to help turn on a light within the consciousness of humanity, to help all souls who read it awaken to a deeper understanding of their relationship to the Divine. In reading this book, you are engaging with Divine energies that have been sent across time and space to anyone who has chosen to engage this book and all that it offers. You may feel these transmissions now as you are reading, or they may be more subtle, showing up as changes in your life that happen slowly over time once you have engaged with this book fully.

Origins

This book was born out of a series of mystical awakenings that happened to me beginning in January 2007, when I was traveling in Laos, and which continued for many months, into October 2007.

The first of these mystical experiences was a vision I had of Mikao Usui, the late founder of the energetic healing system known as Reiki. I had this vision while in the small, beautiful Laotian city of Luang Prabang, a city that was once the royal capitol of Laos and is still known for the splendor of its many Buddhist temples. In this vision, Usui placed a ball of white light into my heart. He told me that the time had come for Reiki to evolve into a system far beyond what it was, that Reiki would be key to a wave of human awakening that was going to sweep the planet. After this visionary empowerment from Reiki's late founder, I felt a deeper connection to all things, a sense of unity with the Divine far beyond anything I had known before. Shortly after this experience, new Reiki symbols for forgiveness and karmic release were revealed to me, symbols that were powerful and effective and which are revealed later in this book. Other mystical occurrences happened at this time in my life as well, things that some may think were hallucinations but which, to me, were the opening of a doorway to the Divine. Complex mathematical equations would at times appear before me, equations that my rational mind could not understand but which made me feel ecstatic when contemplating them. I began sensing eternity, having what Buddhists call a satori experience, wherein the illusions of time and separateness fall away and all that is left is the Divine, never-ending magic that is the root of all that exists.

These satori experiences I was having were not induced by rituals or chemical substances but instead were happening spontaneously, almost daily over a number of weeks. Accompanying these awakening experiences were also teachings of how the Reiki system of energy healing could be both simplified and expanded. The book I was writing at the time, *The Reiki Magic Guide to Self-Attunement*, was undergoing the last stages of the editorial process before going to print, and it was clearly too late to include these new teachings in that book. So I began compiling these teachings with the sense that they were a new and important aspect of the evolution of Reiki as a system of healing. What I did not fully understand at first was that these new tools were much more than an expansion of Reiki as a system of healing: they were, in fact, new Reiki tools to open the door to spiritual awakening.

Reiki and Spirituality

Reiki is an energy healing system. In this book, Reiki is updated and focused in order to promote a deeper sense of spiritual awakening by stripping away some of the karmic debris that prevents us from seeing our own true Divine nature. The Reiki techniques in this book are mostly new and extremely powerful. Be ready to engage real change in your life if you decide to work with these new Reiki tools.

I offer the following chapters of this book as a path of healing and spiritual awakening. It is not the only path, but it is one that is simple, accessible, and already in your hands. I know that in this age of crisis, one of the solutions is for us as a species to take ownership of our spiritual heritage, of the deep connection with the Divine that exists within all of us.

I believe that by embracing our deepest connection with the Divine, and knowing that we are inseparable from it, we will come to naturally resolve the many problems our planet faces, from ecological holocaust to economic injustice, from mass starvation in some parts of the world to genocide in others. We are at the precipice of either a new beginning or a dreadful demise. My hope is that this book, and others like it, will help tip the balance in favor of the delightful outcome: one of spiritual bliss for the billions of people who live on this planet and an awakening to the majesty of all life itself.

1

THE REIKI STAIRWAY
TO HEAVEN

*A Reiki energy transmission has been sent
to all who read this chapter. As you read,
Reiki is being sent to you to further cleanse
your system and take you deeper into a
space of communion with the Divine.*

Reiki is a form of Divine energy healing. The word *Reiki* literally translates from Japanese as "Universal Life Force." This system of healing was discovered around the turn of the previous century by a Japanese mystic named Mikao Usui, who lived from 1865 to 1926. Since its discovery, Reiki has grown to be perhaps the world's most popular form of energetic healing, and yet the deeper potential for Reiki as a system of spiritual awakening has, in many ways, remained untapped.

The Five Principles
There is written evidence that Mikao Usui was interested in Reiki as a path not only for healing but also for spiritual awakening. In his teachings, he offered five principles of Reiki that embody an awakened spiritual point of view for being and living in the world. Though translations of these principles can be found in numerous books and on many websites, each with its own interpretation of the principles, all of the translations express the importance of a daily practice of transcending anger, letting go of worry, expressing gratitude, honoring all life, and

living and working with integrity. Following is my own interpretation of
the many available translations of Usui's Five Principles of Reiki:

> *Just for today, I forgive all sources of anger.*
> *Just for today, I release all worry.*
> *Just for today, I live with gratitude.*
> *Just for today, I am kind to all living things.*
> *Just for today, I am honest in all that I do.*

As these principles show, the original goal of Reiki was not just
physical or emotional healing; it was meant to guide a person who
wishes to follow a spiritual path. Many Reiki Masters still teach Usui's
Five Principles, but too often that is where the spiritual aspect of the
Reiki teaching ends.

It is my belief that Usui's Reiki principles actually point to the possibility of how deeply Reiki can impact and change our lives: that Reiki
can, in fact, be a doorway to spiritual awakening, to realizing that place
of *no separation* between you and the Divine, and that Divine essence
that is in all things. Unfortunately, until recently there have been few
specific Reiki techniques that actually address the deep karmic issues
that prevent us from fully living Usui's Five Principles of Reiki. These
issues occur because we are too lost in the consciousness of separation
to keep our hearts open; Reiki can be used to heal those spiritual issues
and open our lives to the Divine.

Reiki Training

Throughout 2007, I was shown new Reiki techniques that allow Usui's
original spiritual intent for Reiki to be realized. The new Reiki empowerments and techniques laid out in this book are not intended as a Reiki
certification program, nor as a replacement for proven Reiki healing
techniques. The empowerments and techniques here are supplemental
to the Reiki system and allow both the layperson and the trained Reiki
practitioner to use Reiki as a path to spiritual awakening. Though this
book does provide some wonderful new Reiki tools that can be adapted
for personal healing, my goal in writing this book is to reclaim Reiki as
a path for spiritual awakening. Those wishing to learn more about Reiki

for the purpose of physical or emotional healing should either get professional Reiki training from a certified Reiki Master or read my previous book, *The Reiki Magic Guide to Self-Attunement*, which will allow you to attune yourself to all levels of Reiki, including the Master level.

For those reading this book who are untrained in the Reiki system and who simply seek a path to spiritual awakening, you should find it easy to read and use this work without the knowledge of the many symbols, hand positions, and degrees of Reiki that are necessary when using Reiki as a healing system. I have found that, as important as such things are to Reiki as a healing system, they can be bypassed when using Reiki as a system of spiritual awakening. And for those who are already trained in Reiki, please know that the techniques in this book are not intended to replace or challenge your own training as a Reiki healer but simply to offer new techniques for using Reiki as a path to spiritual awakening.

Working with the Higher Self

Most of the techniques in this book expand on the new paradigm within the Reiki lineage of working collaboratively with the Higher Self. When working with the Higher Self, you can send multiple Reiki treatments across many lifetimes simultaneously. Also, Reiki at the level of the Higher Self becomes more malleable and can be shaped into wonderful energy devices, such as Reiki Halos, Reiki Pyramids, and Reiki Holograms. These energy devices help to facilitate intensive karmic release, which can lead to spiritual awakening. It is also possible with these Higher Self techniques to use Reiki as though it were a small laser. I call this energy device a Reiki Cord, and it can be created and infused across the time line of your many lives in order to clear away karmic debris at the moment it was created.

Open Yourself to New Views

Numerous tools are offered in the following chapters, and the one theme underlying all of them is that Reiki is a far more expansive system than was previously known. And if you embrace that expanded point of view, many things become possible, even the awakening of that veil of Maya within your own energy system that holds you in a consciousness of separation from the Divine. Once that veil is awakened, the individual melts back into the awareness that all things are One. It is with that intention of helping individuals melt back into the One that these new Reiki techniques have arisen. It is my hope that these new tools will be taken for what they are: not a replacement for traditional methods of Reiki healing, but an open door into a new world, a magical world where Reiki is a path to spiritual awakening.

2

THE FIRST EMPOWERMENT: STEPPING ON THE REIKI STAIRWAY TO HEAVEN

A Reiki energy transmission has been sent to all who read this chapter. As you read, Reiki is being sent to you to further awaken your system and take you deeper into a space of communion with the Divine.

Awakening is when you empty from the dream that has held your consciousness hostage and open your eyes to what truly is. The mad fibers of the imagination no longer rule your psyche, and your emotions are no longer ruled by the illusory world of the phantoms created by your own mind. Most of humanity is existing in a dream, a dream that either says Divinity does not exist or that the Divine is something separate from us. Such a dream leads to a separation consciousness, a consciousness that says we are impermanent and fleeting, at times giving us the sense that life itself has no meaning.

Spiritual Awakening

When you awaken spiritually, you see that the Divine is in everything, including yourself. As you deepen into that awareness of your own Divinity, that eternal presence within you, you see and feel that presence in all things. It is one eternal presence. The Divine presence is an eternal laugh emanating from all creation, a laughter that exists within you and engulfs everything around you. It is the laughter of the Divine, amused at its own eternal game of hide-and-seek with itself. On some level, awakening spiritually is nothing more than playing peekaboo with God and learning how to see God everywhere, including—and perhaps most importantly—within yourself.

Many paths can lead to spiritual awakening. In recent human history, some of the more direct paths have come to us as bands of heavenly light that emanate directly from the Divine. These bands of light are Deeksha, Reiki, and other energy systems, and they can help us to awaken from the dream that we are separate from the Divine.

Understanding the Dream of Separation

I believe that the dream of separation is the primary source of most human suffering. Only when we come to live the ancient Sanskrit adage *Tat tvam asi*, which translates as "That otherness is myself," will we begin to reap the harvest from the concepts that constitute our society, such as personal freedom, abundance, and the pursuit of happiness, concepts that come more from a Western social perspective based on individuality as opposed to Oneness.

When you recognize that the part of you that is eternal and infinite exists in another, you are less likely to feel afraid of that other or feel alone. The same is true on the larger scale: when we as a species come to realize that our fellow creatures on this Earth are extensions of ourselves, then we will begin to treat the planet with infinitely more respect than we did in the twentieth century.

To begin our journey as a species toward awakening, it is important that we first embrace the unifying energy that binds us all together. We are all from the same One, no matter what name you give it. Jesus implied as much when he said to treat others as you would treat yourself. The Buddhist text the *Diamond Sutra* refers to it as seeing all existence as part of the universal diamond. Many religions make mention of this concept that, in truth, there is no separation and there is no hierarchy in receiving the blessings of Heaven. In Judaism, one of the great prayers is "Hear O Israel, the Lord is our God. The Lord is One." In other words, if the Lord is One, there is no two, no three, no four, nothing other than the Oneness that is God. Understanding this intellectually is not so difficult. Even science says that all the universe comes from One, a single event called the Big Bang.

Empowering All That We Are with Divine Energy

There is a deep difference between understanding something intellectually and understanding something within your body, your psyche, and your spirit. My work as an energy healer has taught me that energy work enters the cells of the physical body, enters the emotional body, and enters the subconscious. Energy work helps to release karmic conditioning, which can keep a person blinded to the truth that we are all part of God and Goddess, the Great Divine, that we are nothing other than a portion of Divine Consciousness that has chosen to forget itself as Divine for the purpose of playing a game called life.

Let us begin our journey toward awakening with the series of empowerments I call the Reiki Stairway to Heaven. Once this series of empowerments is complete, you will have the tools necessary to begin the path of your own spiritual awakening. These empowerments are new to the Reiki lineage, so they may be unfamiliar to those already trained as Reiki healers. However, the doorway that opens when you receive this series of empowerments leads to a path of spiritual awakening.

Please note that these empowerments should not be engaged in all at once. Instead, they should be spread out over a period of weeks or, in some cases, even longer. Reiki is a wonderful spiritual tool, but these empowerments could be overwhelming if you were to receive all of them simultaneously or even within the same week. This is because with each Reiki empowerment, your entire energy system will be changed forever, raising your vibration to a higher level. And each time your vibration changes, changes will occur in your life. Therefore, please use a steady and cautious pace when engaging the Reiki empowerments.

The First Empowerment

The first empowerment in this process is for both your physical form and your Higher Self. The spiritual aspect of the empowerment makes it unique and offers you the ability to transcend Reiki as simply a healing modality and use Reiki instead as a tool for spiritual awakening. The empowerment itself is sent via a Reiki chant to all who willingly say the chant with the intent of being empowered with the Reiki energy.

When you are ready to receive the Reiki empowerment, I recommend that you first take a bath with a pinch of sea salt. This cleanses your aura and also symbolizes your rebirth into a new paradigm of setting out on a journey of spiritual awakening. Afterward, I recommend lighting a white candle to Mikao Usui and those beings who have brought the gift of Reiki to humanity. Do this just prior to saying the chant.

The Energy Exchange

Traditionally, Reiki also requires an exchange of energy. Usually, that would mean paying money or bartering with the Reiki Master who is empowering you with the Reiki energy. But in this case, because I am not taking from my personal time to teach each individual who asks to receive a Reiki empowerment from this book, I recommend that you offer at least three hours of your time and energy to a worthy cause for each level of Reiki empowerment you receive from this book. You could volunteer for a charity, or you could use your Reiki skills to benefit a friend, humanity, or the planet as a whole. A technique on how to use Reiki in this manner is in the following chapter.

Once you have meditated on what your offering back to the greater good should be, please commit to that Reiki energy exchange. My experience is that those who try to bypass this important exchange eventually do not reap the full benefits of their new Reiki gifts. It is not that they will not be empowered with Reiki, but that they will not spiritually *own* the power of this new gift and thus will be less likely to use it with wisdom and clarity for their own spiritual evolution toward awakening.

Preparing for and Activating the First Empowerment

Having decided what your exchange will be, take the sea salt bath. Afterward, dress yourself in a manner that suits the occasion. This is an important ceremony. And make sure that you light a white candle to honor the Reiki lineage, including Mikao Usui, the founder of Reiki, as part of this sacred ceremony.

Once you have made all the necessary preparations, ask to receive the first of the Reiki empowerments by saying the following:

> *Blessed are those who have brought us Reiki*
> *Blessed are those who continue this sacred light*
> *I and my Higher Self*
> *ask for the first empowerment of Reiki*
> *Blessings unto all*
> *Blessings unto me*

While saying the chant, you may feel lightheaded. Or you may feel love surrounding you as the empowerment merges with your energy system. Or you may feel little or even nothing at all. People's experiences of the empowerment vary. It is important, however, to treat this time as sacred and offer yourself the quiet time to melt in with this new loving energy that will be with you for the rest of your life. You might want to take a walk in the woods or do something special for yourself on this wonderful day. Whatever you decide to do, know that the changes that come with this new energy gift are life altering. You have taken a giant and eternal step forward on your path of spiritual awakening.

3

THE STEP OF DAILY REIKI TREATMENTS FOR SPIRITUAL AWAKENING

A Divine energy transmission for releasing
obstacles on your spiritual path has been
sent to all who read this chapter.

The purpose of this book is to offer a path of spiritual awakening. There are many uses for Reiki. This book focuses on Reiki for spiritual awakening.

Gaining Access to Your Higher Self

To use Reiki after your first empowerment for spiritual awakening, it is best to ask your Higher Self to run Reiki directly into any karmic or spiritual blocks that need to be released in order for your awakening to occur. Traditionally, there would be no hand position for engaging this kind of issue with Reiki at this level. Though Reiki has always been able to bring about profound spiritual change, such change was often seen more as a byproduct of cumulative Reiki sessions than as something that could be addressed through direct and specific techniques. Now, because we are working with the wisdom of your Higher Self—the core essence and most Divine aspect of your spiritual being—it is possible to use Higher Self Reiki techniques to send this energy wherever it needs to go. And, because your Higher Self exists beyond time and space, and has access to all of your lifetimes, it is even possible for this level of Reiki treatment to work on more than one lifetime simultaneously.

Whenever I am working with my Higher Self, I call it Sahu, an ancient Egyptian term for the Higher Self. I began doing this in the late 1990s, when I was first starting to experiment with Reiki and other energy practices. I still use the term *Sahu* for my own personal Reiki practice but have found recently that any word referring to the Higher Self will suffice as long as the intention is to connect and work with the most Divine and timeless aspect of your own being.

Offering Energy to Complete the Task

Working with the Higher Self also requires an offering of energy to the Higher Self for it to complete the task that has been requested. There are a number of ways to do this. For me, the simplest way is to offer three breaths to my Higher Self, which uses the life energy of each of those breaths to activate my request. So when I make a verbal request, I blow three times at the end.

Reiki Treatment for Spiritual Awakening

To begin a Reiki treatment for spiritual awakening, find a time and place where you can relax and fully integrate the experience. One suggestion is to do this just before going to bed, as sleeping and dreaming can often be the perfect format for working through and integrating deep releases at the karmic and spiritual level. If you prefer to engage the treatment while awake, then I recommend giving yourself at least an hour after the treatment for integration. It is best to engage the treatment while lying down, as often the treatment will take you into a place of deep relaxation.

Once you have found an appropriate place to lie down and receive the treatment, speak the following chant:

By the power of the golden light within
By the power of the sacred breath
I manifest this truth
I now will my Higher Self to send a one-hour Reiki treatment
to all of my bodies in all of my lifetimes
for release of karmic and spiritual blockages
I manifest this now
So be it!

(Blow three times.)

Now, relax and let the Reiki treatment envelop your entire being. Because hand positions do not need to be specific, given that your Higher Self is weaving this treatment in the most effective way possible, simply place your hands anywhere on your body as the treatment is continuing. The added warmth of Reiki flowing through your hands and into your body is comforting. And unlike traditional Reiki, you are free to put your hands wherever you wish.

This treatment can be repeated as often as you like. It will help to loosen energetic debris being held within any of your energetic bodies, debris that needs to be released for your spiritual awakening to occur.

Higher Self Reiki Treatment for Specific Situations

You can also use this same technique to send Reiki energy to a good cause as part of your energy exchange for receiving the Reiki empowerment. Following is a template chant you can use for sending Reiki in any number of situations:

By the power of the golden light within
By the power of the sacred breath
I manifest this truth
I now will my Higher Self to send a one-hour Reiki treatment
to [specific situation]
I manifest this now
So be it!

(Blow three times.)

Remember that keeping your commitment to an energy exchange is essential to *owning* your new Reiki abilities. So please use the preceding treatment option for sending at least three hours of Reiki to good causes, unless you have decided upon other energy exchanges that do not involve sending Reiki.

Use this new tool for your spiritual journey by sending yourself the Reiki treatment for spiritual awakening every day. It may be best if you do this at a regular time each day so that you have a routine that you can easily organize your life around. Personally, I invoke this treatment before going to bed. But do what works for you, as long as you commit to making it a daily practice. After twenty-one days, you will have cleared a great deal of karmic debris from your energy system and will be ready for the second empowerment on the Reiki Stairway to Heaven.

4

THE SECOND EMPOWERMENT: STEPPING IT UP

*A Divine energy treatment to help release negative
karmic conditioning has been sent across time
and space to all who read this chapter.*

The second empowerment of Reiki will deepen your relationship with
Reiki. This empowerment corresponds energetically with the Second
Degree Reiki attunement that is taught in the traditional Reiki system.
However, with the new Higher Self Reiki techniques and the focus
on spiritual awakening, there is no specific need to fully engage the
Reiki symbols that are traditionally taught at this level. I will include
these symbols in the following chapter out of respect for the Reiki
lineage and so that you do have an understanding of them and their
meanings, but the Higher Self Reiki techniques do not require their use.

The Second Energy Exchange

As with the first Reiki empowerment, you are likely to undergo some
changes in the weeks that follow. And, in keeping with the concept of an
energy exchange, you should meditate on what you wish to give back
to the Divine in exchange for this wonderful spiritual gift. I recommend
offering at least three hours of Reiki to some worthy cause, using the
technique shown in the previous chapter. Let your own intuition be your
guide, but offer a significant amount of time to give back to the common
good in exchange for this precious gift you are about to receive.

Preparing for and Activating the Second Empowerment

Once you have decided on and committed to the energy exchange, and have again made time for yourself to be in sacred space during this sacred process, take a bath with a pinch of sea salt in it for cleansing your aura. Then, dress in a ritual manner that, for you, honors the sacredness of what you are about to embark upon in engaging the second Reiki empowerment. As before, I recommend lighting a white candle to the Divine and Mikao Usui to honor this sacred process.

Once you have completed your meditation on the energy exchange and prepared yourself with the cleansing bath and ritual dress, you can engage the Reiki chant that follows. It will empower you to experience Reiki at a deeper level than ever before.

Blessed are those who have brought us Reiki
Blessed are those who continue this sacred light
I and my Higher Self
Ask for the second empowerment of Reiki
Blessings unto all
Blessings unto me

Allow your consciousness to linger quietly in the upgraded spiritual vibration that you have just attained. Be still. Notice the feelings that emerge from having engaged this sacred empowerment. Take time for yourself to honor this day. Treat it almost as you would a birthday. Maybe take yourself out for a fine dinner. Or write a poem to God. Do something to celebrate—yes, celebrate—the wondrous being that is you. For that you, as you will know by the end of this book, is also the Divine, an inseparable and infinite piece of God and Goddess. Cherish it! Love it! Be kind to it and treat it with reverence. And know that nothing you ever did in this life or any other can diminish the eternal link you have with the Divine. For it and you are the same.

LIFTING UP YOUR MIND ON THE REIKI STAIRWAY TO HEAVEN

A Divine energy transmission for spiritual integration has been sent across time and space to all who read this chapter.

The purpose of this book is spiritual awakening, and the focus of this chapter is on techniques that will enhance your journey of spiritual awakening. Reiki is a wonderful energy healing system with a variety of techniques and purposes. As I noted earlier, some aspects of that system are not included in this text in order to keep the focus primarily on spiritual awakening.

Traditionally, the Reiki empowerment that you received in the previous chapter would activate your ability to use the first three Reiki symbols. And though the Higher Self Reiki techniques for spiritual awakening bypass many of those symbols' traditional functions, it is still important to know and understand these symbols, to take your consciousness deeply into them and their power, which you are using via a simplified Higher Self Reiki technique.

Cho Ku Rei

The first of these symbols is called Cho Ku Rei. It is used to increase the flow of Reiki. Traditionally, you would specifically memorize how it is drawn. For our purposes, you simply need to have an awareness of what it looks like and what it is used for. Your Higher Self will do the rest of the work when invoking this symbol by name.

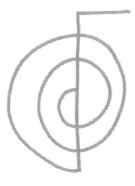

Cho Ku Rei

Sei He Ki

The second Reiki symbol is Sei He Ki and is used primarily for mental and emotional healing. This symbol can be an important part of the spiritual awakening process. Certain uses of this symbol will be invoked by your Higher Self by name for awakening deeper into a place of Oneness with the Divine. Sei He Ki can also be used for protection.

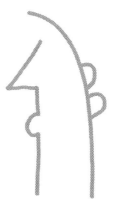

Sei He Ki

Hon Sha Ze Sho Nen

The third Reiki symbol is known as Hon Sha Ze Sho Nen. The primary purpose of this symbol is to send Reiki to distant points across time and space. Because your Higher Self transcends time and space, it can send Reiki without invoking the Hon Sha Ze Sho Nen symbol. However, there are some more esoteric uses of this symbol, which will be explained in later chapters. For now, look at it with reverence, knowing that it will be an important part of your journey into spiritual awakening.

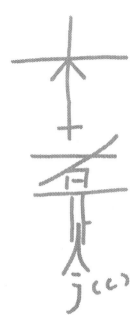

Hon Sha Ze Sho Nen

Using the Second Reiki Empowerment

The great psychologist Carl Jung once said, "Enlightenment is not imagining figures of light but making the darkness conscious." To me, that is one of the most important statements ever made. Some New Age circles cherish the belief that you can imagine yourself into heaven simply by always visualizing the positive. But true spiritual awakening requires that you shed the karmic and spiritual obstacles that have become a part of your energetic system due to the actions and beliefs that have been imprinted upon you over many lifetimes. By working on deeper issues—

karmic and spiritual issues—you can focus the spiritual light of Reiki on those places of darkness, those places where you are spiritually asleep, and awaken them. Now, let us begin the work of using this new level of Reiki empowerment to deepen your connection with the Divine.

Your Higher Self now has the ability to send multiple Reiki treatments through many lifetimes and focus on the deeper mental and emotional issues that have created the karmic veil between you and your own Divine nature. The ability of the Higher Self to send Reiki to these root causes of karmic and spiritual issues is endless.

Following is a Higher Self Reiki chant to deepen your connection with the Divine by bringing light to those areas in your psyche where you have been spiritually asleep for many lifetimes:

> *By the power of the golden light within*
> *By the power of the sacred breath*
> *I manifest this truth*
> *I now will my Higher Self*
> *to send a one-hour Sei He Ki mental/emotional Reiki treatment*
> *to all of my lifetimes*
> *to any point in space and time*
> *where I have encouraged the illusion of separation from the Divine*
> *I manifest this now*
> *So be it!*

(Blow three times.)

This one treatment, when repeated daily over a number of weeks, will loosen the roots of separation consciousness, that aspect of consciousness that believes itself to be separate from the Divine. The positive effects will bleed into your daily life, into your dreams, and into all that you are. And eventually, when used in conjunction with your other tools for spiritual awakening, it will help release you from the dream of separation from the Divine. I recommend using this treatment every day for three weeks before moving on to the next empowerment of the Reiki Stairway to Heaven.

THE THIRD EMPOWERMENT: LEAPING UP THE STAIRWAY

A Divine energy transmission focused on deep spiritual integration has been sent across time and space to all who read this chapter.

The third Reiki empowerment, sent through the chant revealed later in this chapter, is the most empowering gift you will have received so far in the spiritual journey provided through these pages. It will change your life in profound ways, even if you never use the gift of Reiki again. It will shift your vibration to a new and higher level, a level that will refine your soul. It will also, when combined with the other Higher Self Reiki techniques, accelerate your process of spiritual awakening.

Spiritual Metamorphosis and Embracing the New You

Engage this chant with the wisdom and understanding that you are undergoing a spiritual metamorphosis. You, like the caterpillar that becomes a butterfly, will dissolve and be re-formed into something magical and new. Step into this chant knowing and owning the changes that are to come. Make certain that your energy exchange with the Divine is equal to the gift that you are about to receive. You may want to donate time each week sending Reiki to a good cause using the techniques in chapter 3. Or, if you have money to spare, you might want to offer money to a charitable cause as your energy exchange. In the end, the exchange has to feel right to you. Only by committing to a significant offering to the Divine through some act of good works will you be able to truly own the power of your new spiritual gift.

Treat This Day as Holy

Once you have committed to your energy exchange with the Divine, set aside a full day for the experience of the attunement. You will want to take your aura-cleansing bath with a pinch of sea salt and dress appropriately for the ceremonial occasion. Because this empowerment goes far deeper than any of the previous ones in this book, create an altar for the occasion as well. Place a white candle honoring the Divine and Mikao Usui on the altar. You may want to add flowers to your altar, pictures of saints, drawings of angels, or other touches to note the significance of this occasion.

When you are ready, speak the Reiki empowerment chant that follows:

Blessed are those who have brought us Reiki
Blessed are those who continue this sacred light
I and my Higher Self
ask for the third empowerment of Reiki
Blessings unto all
Blessings unto me

Take time to appreciate the spiritual energies that surround and engulf you during this attunement. You may want to spend the remainder of this day in meditation or take a long walk in the woods. Treat this day as holy by acknowledging it with some special activity after the attunement. Whether you sit quietly in meditation or treat yourself to a massage, do something that works for you to acknowledge this as a special day in your life, a day that will change your life forever.

RISING UP FROM THE
PLACE OF YOUR SOUL

*A Reiki treatment for awakening at the
soul level has been sent across time and
space to all who read this chapter.*

The third Reiki empowerment for spiritual awakening is equal to
that of the Master level in traditional Reiki. And though this is not
a Reiki certification program, and you are not being taught how to
teach and train others in the Reiki system, you now have access to energies that can reshape you at the core soul level. Traditionally, these
energies are focused more on physical healing and less on spiritual
awakening. Because this book is about spiritual awakening, the following techniques will be focused on that purpose. I encourage you to
experiment with the techniques that follow and to adapt them to your
own journey of awakening, however your path extends through the
world of spirit.

You now have access to three more Reiki symbols because of the
third Reiki empowerment. And though you will not engage these symbols as directly as you would when using traditional Reiki techniques,
knowing them and extending your consciousness into them is essential
for deepening your process of using Reiki for spiritual awakening. These
three symbols are the Tibetan Master symbol, the Usui Master symbol,
and a symbol called Raku.

Both of the Master symbols are referred to as Dia-Ko-Myo, which my Reiki Master, Mary Dudek, once told me means, "Great Being of the Universe, shine on me, be my friend." Whether this translation is linguistically correct or not, I have found that it does reflect how the Master symbols feel energetically: they open up the entire universe to embrace you from a place of friendship.

The Tibetan Master Symbol

The Tibetan Master symbol can deepen the flow of Reiki, and it allows Reiki to work on a *soul level*. It is also an important symbol used in Reiki initiations, though for the purpose of this book you will be using it only for its deepening and soul-level effect.

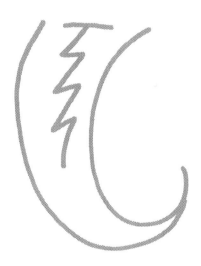

Tibetan Master (Dia-Ko-Myo)

The Usui Master Symbol

The Usui Master symbol also deepens the flow of Reiki, and, like the Tibetan Master symbol, it focuses Reiki to work on a soul level. Essentially, it can be used interchangeably with the Tibetan Master symbol and is also an important symbol used in Reiki initiations. Some Reiki traditions use one symbol or the other for Reiki initiations, and others use both symbols. And though this book does not engage the traditional Reiki initiation process, I include both of these symbols for taking your consciousness deeper into the Reiki lineage.

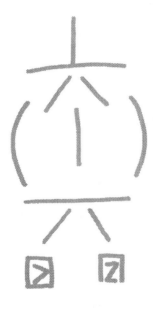

Usui Master (Dia-Ko-Myo)

The Raku Symbol

The Raku symbol has only one primary purpose in Reiki, which is to open the aura during the Reiki initiation process. I offer it here to facilitate the deepening of your consciousness into the Reiki lineage.

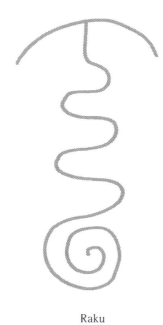

Raku

Using the Third Reiki Empowerment

Now that you know about the additional Reiki symbols that have been activated within your energy system by the third Reiki empowerment, begin to use the awesome awakening potential of this empowerment by sending a Reiki treatment to your own soul. Following is a Higher Self Reiki technique that you can use daily to accelerate the process of awakening at the soul level.

By the power of the golden light within
By the power of the sacred breath
I manifest this truth
I now will my Higher Self
to send a one-hour Dia-Ko-Myo Reiki treatment to my soul
for accelerating the process of spiritual awakening
I manifest this now
So be it!

(Blow three times.)

This treatment can affect your soul in a variety of ways. Personally, I have found it to have a very cleansing effect, as if it purifies my being down to the very core. Know that by using this treatment daily you are bathing your soul in a powerful Divine light, a light that encourages you to see the Divine as a dear and close friend. Make a commitment to use this treatment daily, preferably just before going to bed. Notice the impact that it has on your dreams, on your attitude, and, eventually, on how you see yourself in relationship with the Divine.

STEPPING INTO INFINITY WITH THE UNIVERSAL REIKI HEALING GRID

*A Divine energy treatment for releasing
the illusory veil of separation has been
sent to all who read this chapter.*

The concept of a Reiki Grid is not a new one. For years, Reiki practitioners have used crystals empowered with Reiki to create grids that are energetically charged for various healing purposes. These grids are fueled by the energy of Reiki embedded in each crystal.

How the Universal Reiki Healing Grid Was Created

In my experiments with Reiki at the Higher Self level, I was eventually shown by the spirit of Mikao Usui how to work on the Higher Self level to manifest Reiki Grids on a more universal scale. These grids are permanent, and anyone who is attuned to Reiki and has knowledge of these grids can gain access to them. The first grid is the Universal Reiki Healing Grid. It was created in the spring of 2007 in collaboration with the Deva (or Divine Intelligence) of Reiki, the Deva of all the celestial bodies (planets and stars) in this universe, the spirit of Mikao Usui, and my Higher Self. If you could see the Universal Reiki Healing Grid, it would appear as bands of Reiki that link each and every celestial body in the universe. These bands of light work harmoniously to form the Universal

29

Reiki Healing Grid and are permanently available as a healing device for all who wish to use them for the highest good.

Invoking and Using the Universal Reiki Healing Grid

The Universal Reiki Healing Grid can be used for a variety of purposes. But because the intent of this book is to help humanity awaken to a deeper relationship with the Divine, the following techniques have awakening as their primary goal. Following are a series of invocations you can use to gain access to the Universal Reiki Healing Grid and to deepen your spiritual journey of awakening.

The following invocation works primarily on healing any separation consciousness held within your energy system. It does this by immersing you in the Universal Reiki Healing Grid, which connects all things. Use it as frequently as needed, particularly on those days when you feel angry or upset or are creating an *us versus them* mentality that causes a sense of separation.

By the power of the golden light within
By the power of the sacred breath
I manifest this truth
I now will my Higher Self
to immerse me into the Universal Reiki Healing Grid for the next hour
to work on healing all separation consciousness in my energy system
I manifest this now
So be it!

(Blow three times.)

The wonderful thing about the Universal Reiki Healing Grid is that it is powerful enough to effect real change and yet gentle enough that you tend to remain fully conscious and can go about other tasks during your day while the Universal Reiki Healing Grid is doing its work. Though I would not use this technique while driving a car or operating dangerous machinery, I do often use it while I am at the office. And though I may be aware of a tingling sensation as the grid is working on an issue for me, it is not so intense as to distract me from the task at hand.

Because part of the path of spiritual awakening has to do with healing relationships between you and your parents, family members, friends, and significant other, a wonderful way to use this grid is to have it work on a situation between you and somebody else. Understand that the grid is not sending Reiki to the other person or persons but is instead working to smooth out any misunderstandings or negative energies between you. It is not a cure-all but can work as a wonderful salve for many life situations, especially when repeated over a period of time.

The template that follows can be used to help bring healing to any situation; adapt the wording as needed:

> *By the power of the golden light within*
> *By the power of the sacred breath*
> *I manifest this truth*
> *I now will my Higher Self*
> *to immerse the situation between me and [person or situation]*
> *into the Universal Reiki Healing Grid for the next hour*
> *to work on healing [issue]*
> *I manifest this now*
> *So be it!*

(Blow three times.)

By helping to heal some of the situations in your life that need healing, the grid helps you to see some of the karmic patterns that are the root cause of such issues. You can use this on something as simple as smoothing out a minor disagreement with your significant other or on something as difficult as a long-term issue, such as having been abused as a child. I use the Universal Reiki Healing Grid daily, for easing the small issues that arise on the job as well as for working on deeper issues as they arise in the path of my own spiritual growth.

The infinite nature of this grid, which stretches across the universe as bands of light among the stars and planets, makes my day-to-day life easier. The grid allows me to focus on my own connection with the Divine while I immerse my cares in the grid. I encourage you to use this grid often. Let it serve you in your awakening to your own connection with the One.

THE UNIVERSAL REIKI INTEGRATION GRID, THE HANDRAIL OF THE STAIRWAY

A Divine energy transmission focused on deep spiritual integration has been sent across time and space to all who read this chapter.

Did you ever run up a stairway as a child, with your hands in the air, feeling that nothing could stop you, as if you could almost fly? And then suddenly, your foot missed a step, you lost your balance, and you came tumbling down. In my journey as a healer, I have come more and more to see integration as the handrail that keeps us from slipping backward on any healing or spiritual journey. Integration is what keeps us steady and allows us to keep moving forward with the certainty that we won't fall down.

The Creation of a Second Grid

Shortly after my experience of helping bring the Universal Reiki Healing Grid into manifestation, a second universal Reiki Grid was created by a collaboration among my Higher Self and the same beings that helped create the first grid. This grid was shaped and infused with one primary purpose: integration. The Universal Reiki Integration Grid, if you could see it, would look almost exactly like the Universal Reiki Healing Grid, but the bands of Reiki light that compose it are intended only for work on integration.

The Purpose of the Universal Reiki Integration Grid

I offer this tool at this stage of your journey because the steps that follow may begin to strip away some of the core karmic debris and conditioning that has kept you veiled, kept you from knowing your own true Divine nature. This process of lifting the veil is essential to seeing with clarity that eternal Divine presence that is not only you, but everything. And yet this process can, at times, be hard, be disturbing, and make you feel as though the opposite is happening, that you are losing everything that you are. If you begin using the Universal Reiki Integration Grid, it will act like a salve on that process. It will allow you to still feel grounded after very intense energy treatments. It will keep your mind focused when the very core of your being is undergoing a metamorphosis.

If you think of spiritual awakening as being like the caterpillar becoming the butterfly, one thing you must know about caterpillars is that they become deconstructed while in the cocoon. Essentially, the Universal Reiki Integration Grid allows you to remain calm and centered while the illusion of your own separateness from the Divine is deconstructed by the energy work laid out in the following chapters.

Invoking the Universal Reiki Integration Grid

To have your Higher Self immerse you in the Universal Reiki Integration Grid, say the following invocation:

By the power of the golden light within
By the power of the sacred breath
I manifest this truth
I now will my Higher Self
to immerse me into the Universal Reiki Integration Grid
for the next hour
I manifest this now
So be it!

(Blow three times.)

You can always adjust the time that you want to be immersed in the Universal Reiki Integration Grid. You can make it longer or shorter than the hour specified in the invocation. But because you have already gone up several steps of the Reiki Stairway to Heaven, and have already received some life-changing empowerments, it might be time to take hold of the handrail. And you can do so now by giving yourself the luxury of integrating at a deeper level by engaging in a full hour of being immersed in the Universal Reiki Integration Grid. Do so before going to sleep and see how you feel the following morning. It will prepare you for the deeper releases yet to come in the following chapters.

10

ESCALATING AWAKENING WITH THE UNIVERSAL OMEGA REIKI GRID

A Divine energy transmission focused on
deep karmic release has been sent across
time and space to all who read this chapter.

Like the other universal Reiki Grids, the Universal Omega Reiki Grid was created in collaboration with the Deva of Reiki, the Deva of all the celestial bodies in the universe, the spirit of Mikao Usui, and my Higher Self. It exists as bands of Divine light across the heavens, which link the celestial bodies. Of the three grids, this one is the most powerful and the one that, with consistent use, will bring about the most change.

The Meaning of Omega

The term *Omega* has shown up in my life with respect to healing in a number of ways. I live and work at the Omega Institute, a holistic center named after a concept of the Jesuit mystic Teilhard de Chardin. His idea is that the Omega point is a place where all consciousness synthesizes into an awareness of itself at all levels. For years at the institute, I taught a meditation class to the staff called Omega Point Meditation. Students would focus their awareness on one single point where all of our consciousnesses intersected and became as One. During these meditations, staff members and I would often have mind-altering experiences, which revealed how deeply interconnected we are at all levels. Years after I began engaging in these meditations, I became a student of Ric Weinman and his own amazing, trademarked form of energy work. I was eventually trained at the fifth level of his system, a level he referred to as Omega, which is one of the highest forms of energy healing I have experienced.

The term *Omega* comes from the ancient Greek alphabet; it is the last letter, the culminating point. When I speak of the Universal Omega Reiki Grid, I am referring to a form of Reiki in which every aspect of the energy is interconnected and aware of both itself and the issues it is working on. It delves into issues at multiple levels of reality simultaneously.

Invoking the Universal Omega Reiki Grid

Use the Universal Omega Reiki Grid for clearing the energy around a relationship, work issue, or other life issue at a core level. Following is a template for using this grid:

> *By the power of the golden light within*
> *By the power of the sacred breath*
> *I manifest this truth*
> *I now will my Higher Self to immerse [person or situation]*
> *in the Universal Omega Reiki Grid*
> *for the next [number] minutes*
> *I manifest this now*
> *So be it!*

(Blow three times.)

Due to the strength of this grid, I tend to use it for only thirty minutes at a time. Also, I recommend following any use of this grid with the Universal Reiki Integration Grid. A general rule of thumb is to use ten minutes in the Universal Reiki Integration Grid for every thirty minutes in the Universal Omega Reiki Grid. This will help rebalance and ground your energy system after the intensity of the Universal Omega Reiki Grid treatment.

When you begin to incorporate this grid into your daily life, everything around you will begin to lighten up. Put situations into the grid and notice how quickly you begin to resolve problems that once seemed unsolvable. This is because the Universal Omega Reiki Grid is a much more powerful tool than anything mentioned in this book so far. You can even put your own journey of awakening into the grid and see what changes come from using the grid in this manner. See how the grid will help to accelerate your journey. The use of this grid has a cumulative effect: the more you use it, the greater impact it will have upon your life.

11

STEPPING INTO FORGIVENESS

A Reiki treatment for forgiveness has been sent
across time and space to all who read this chapter.
While reading this chapter, also imagine forgiv-
ing yourself for anything you have ever done to
harm another, in this or another lifetime.

One of the most powerful tools I was given during a visitation from Mikao Usui in January 2007 was a pair of Reiki symbols for forgiveness. One symbol activates Reiki for self-forgiveness, and the other symbol activates Reiki for forgiving others. The two symbols work by bringing Divine Consciousness directly into the heart, creating a deep spaciousness that allows you to let go of resentment, anger, and other emotions that are often obstacles to forgiveness.

Forgiveness is a concept that at times has been misused to keep people bound to dysfunctional situations. Often, when undergoing my own healing from childhood sexual abuse, I was told by others that I should simply forgive those who abused me. That kind of forgiveness is a lie. It's a way to not deal with the horror of what happened to me. The people who encouraged me to forgive also seemed to not want to hear about or engage any of the facts of what had happened to me during childhood. This misuse of the term *forgiveness*—implying that a person should simply "get over" past wrongs—does not come from a real place, a Divine place. Divine forgiveness does not try to cover up the wound or pretend that it isn't there. Divine forgiveness does something entirely different: it creates an emotional bridge to understanding how and why the events occurred. It also adds a universal sense of compassion for all parties. Instead of sweeping anything under the rug, it brings everything into the light, a light so powerful and compassionate that all wounds are healed in its presence.

The Forgiveness Reiki Symbols

It is this Divine form of forgiveness that is a powerful tool in the process of healing and of spiritual awakening. For me as an energy healer, the following symbols are two of the most precious and useful tools I have come to engage on my spiritual path and my healing path. I call both symbols Forgiveness Reiki symbols, knowing that I use one or the other, or sometimes both, depending on whether I want to forgive myself, another person, or both of us.

Forgiveness Reiki symbol for forgiving yourself

Forgiveness Reiki symbol for forgiving others

Using Forgiveness Reiki

My sense is that two Forgiveness Reiki symbols are necessary because there are subtle differences between forgiving yourself and forgiving someone else. Forgiveness of yourself requires an ownership of having harmed another in some fashion, whether intentionally or unintentionally. When these roles are reversed, you might seek to forgive another. Hence, though both instances are about forgiveness, you play different karmic roles in each. This is why there are two Forgiveness Reiki symbols, not just one.

These symbols are powerful in helping you to release resentment and anger, clearing the path for forgiveness at the deepest root level. At times when you may think that it is not doing anything, you will be surprised to see how this form of Reiki works at all levels. Once I used a combination of these two symbols to send Reiki to a situation in which two other individuals and myself were feeling competitive and jealous. One of the individuals in this triangle seemed to be trying to ruin my relationship with the third individual. I had hoped for a healing of this situation for more than a year, and nothing I had done energetically seemed to have any effect. The three of us lived in the same area and had mutual friends. It was always difficult and uncomfortable when we were all together in the same room. One night, I decided to send a fifteen-minute Forgiveness Reiki treatment to the entire situation, to try to release the karmic baggage that the three of us had accumulated. The next morning, the third person, who had rarely spoken to me for almost a year, showed up and offered a deep and sincere apology. The situation underwent a complete transformation, which I credit to that fifteen-minute Reiki treatment in which I sent forgiveness to the entire situation.

A Reiki empowerment for these two symbols has been sent across time and space to all who say the following chant with the intention of receiving the empowerment. As with the other empowerments in this book, hold an attitude of sacredness toward this empowerment. Take a bath with a pinch of sea salt for cleansing the aura, dress in a manner that is in keeping with the sacredness of the event, and light a white candle to the Divine and Mikao Usui. Also, meditate upon what your energy exchange will be—what good works you will engage in as thanks for receiving the Divine blessing of this empowerment.

Once you have undergone all the ritual aspects and made your commitment for the energy exchange with the Divine, recite the following chant with the intention of being attuned to both symbols of Forgiveness Reiki:

Blessed are those who have brought us Reiki
Blessed are those who continue this sacred light
I and my Higher Self
ask for the empowerment of Forgiveness Reiki
Blessings unto all
Blessings unto me

Take time to let your consciousness linger in these new energetic vibrations. The empowerment of these two symbols will influence your spiritual path but will not involve as large an energetic shift as the previous Reiki empowerments. This is because you have not changed the level of your overall Reiki vibration. You have simply expanded the spectrum of Reiki lights you can access to include the light of Forgiveness Reiki. You may wish to treat this day as a special occasion, just as with the previous empowerments. But because the energetic changes are not as dramatic, I recommend diving directly into the work of forgiveness to deepen your journey toward spiritual awakening.

The Work of Forgiveness
Though most of the techniques in this book bypass the traditional use of Reiki symbols and hand positions, I have found that when using Forgiveness Reiki on yourself, it works best when you place your hand directly over your heart. This is because the heart is where the forgiveness is taking place.

Self-Forgiveness
Start using Forgiveness Reiki by offering a treatment first to yourself. Begin by thinking of something that you have done that you still regret, some action you took or something you said that caused harm to yourself or another. Once you have that situation clearly in mind, visualize the Forgiveness Reiki symbol for forgiving yourself over your palms,

along with the Cho Ku Rei symbol (as seen in chapter 5), which empowers the Forgiveness Reiki symbol to do its job. Now, place your hands over your heart. Begin sending Forgiveness Reiki into your heart by repeating the following:

Cho Ku Rei, Cho Ku Rei, Cho Ku Rei
Forgiveness Reiki, Forgiveness Reiki, Forgiveness Reiki
Cho Ku Rei, Cho Ku Rei, Cho Ku Rei

(Repeat this chant again and again.)

Continue repeating the names of the symbols, and this time mentally picture the event for which you wish to be forgiven, as though you were watching a movie. You may feel your heart become more spacious as an eternal presence may seem to weigh your act against the immensity of time, showing you how small the event actually is when compared with all eternity. Soon, you may notice that even if you try to get angry at yourself about the event, the anger is no longer there: the roots to which it was clinging are now severed, so the anger has nothing to hold onto.

Some issues take only a few minutes to forgive, whereas deeper ones might take quite a bit longer. You can use this technique anytime you want to forgive yourself.

I often use this technique to forgive old wounds I inflicted on other children when I was in school. Because I was growing up in an abusive home, I had a wicked sense of humor and often made fun of other children at school, sometimes causing them to cry. It was my way of escaping my own childhood horror at the time. There is no telling what kind of emotional scars these actions left on these other souls who happened to share the schools and playgrounds with me. Sending Forgiveness Reiki to myself for my actions also, I believe, helps the negativity of these events be released in the psyches of those who suffered from my actions, as we are all interconnected, all One.

I recommend using the Forgiveness Reiki symbol to go through time and clean up any karmic messes you have created, intentionally or unintentionally. Make it part of your daily routine, at least while you are working with this book, to work each day on forgiving yourself for one or more things. You may be surprised at how many things you feel ashamed of once you begin looking at those parts of your life. By using this symbol repeatedly to forgive yourself, you will feel lighter, happier, and more compassionate toward yourself and others.

Forgiving Others

Equally, it is important to use Forgiveness Reiki to activate forgiveness of others in your heart. If you think of all of us as existing in a great karmic playground, then think of resentments as rocks you are intending to throw at others who have hurt you. If all you have is an accumulation of rocks in your pockets, it becomes very hard to play. These rocks can be large or small, filled with harmful intentions or just the thought that justice will pay someone back in the end. In either case, as long as your focus on that playground is on throwing rocks at others, or hoping someone else will throw a rock at them, then it really is hard to simply run, laugh, climb trees, or take on the many other adventures that await us all. For me, forgiveness is emptying your pockets of all those rocks you have been carrying. Even if it might seem like someone deserves payback, it is actually much more liberating to free yourself from having to carry such a load of rocks and to begin seeing the other as simply another child on the Divine playground of life.

To use Forgiveness Reiki for forgiving another, first think of the person you wish to forgive. Then, imagine the Forgiveness Reiki symbol for forgiving others, along with the Cho Ku Rei symbol (as seen in chapter 5), on both of your palms. You are not going to be sending the other person any Reiki at all, for to do so would require their consent and participation. But you are going to be sending Reiki into your own heart, just as you did when forgiving yourself. Now, place your hands over your heart and begin sending Forgiveness Reiki into your heart by repeating the following:

Cho Ku Rei, Cho Ku Rei, Cho Ku Rei
Forgiveness Reiki, Forgiveness Reiki, Forgiveness Reiki
Cho Ku Rei, Cho Ku Rei, Cho Ku Rei

(Repeat this chant again and again, for as long as your intuition tells you to do so.)

While repeating the names of the symbols, and allowing Forgiveness Reiki to flow into your heart, imagine that you are seeing the event that you wish to forgive. It is happening in front of your eyes as though it were a movie. Imagine whomever it is that once harmed you actually playing that harm out again. But this time, be a Divine witness to the event. Keep channeling Forgiveness Reiki into your heart as you do this.

Empowerment through Divine Witness

It might seem cruel to ask you to reimagine a painful event for the purpose of forgiving the one who caused the harm. And if it were not for the fact that Forgiveness Reiki takes you out of the place of victim and into the place of Divine witness, I would agree. But what Forgiveness Reiki actually does is allow you to step out of the victim role and feel free from all cause and effect surrounding the event. Your heart engages that space of eternal spaciousness in which no event, even the most vile, can compare with the infinite and eternal compassion that is held within that sea of forgiveness.

Words do not do this symbol justice, and it is best to simply try it out. I recommend using it on an issue where you feel it is incredibly hard to forgive someone. Try the preceding technique and feel how it frees your heart of the drama, suffering, and cycle of pain that resentment and anger keep you locked into. Forgiveness does not mean that you immediately become good friends with the people you choose to forgive. In many instances, it may be wise for you to never interact with them again, especially in cases of violence or severe abuse. But you can forgive and move on. Returning to the analogy I used before, you can now enjoy the rest of the playground without feeling burdened by all the rocks you were carrying. That does not mean that you should go and play again with bullies, but it does mean that you no longer have to worry or waste your energy on the wish for them to be punished. You can now step away from them, knowing that they are actually just you in disguise, other players in a Divine play. You will also know that nothing you can do to bullies will ever be better than releasing them from their trespasses with the hope that they, too, will one day learn to enjoy the playground for what it truly is: a place of wonder.

Past-Life Forgiveness

You can also work on forgiveness issues for multiple lifetimes by including your Higher Self in the process. Begin by forgiving your own trespasses for all of your lifetimes. Though you will not remember all of these instances, and may not be consciously aware of any of them, start with the assumption that it is very likely that you caused harm to others in your previous lives. Intend that your Higher Self work in conjunction with your subconscious mind, where all of your past-life memories are stored. I recommend using the following invocation just before going to bed so that you will have time for integration as you sleep:

By the power of the golden light within
By the power of the sacred breath
I manifest this truth
I now will my Higher Self to send Forgiveness Reiki for the next hour
through my heart and my subconscious mind
to manifest forgiveness for all of the acts of harm I have caused
to myself or others
in all of my lifetimes
I manifest this now
So be it!

(Blow three times.)

This process is effective and can help restore a sense of innocence and wonder as the karmic baggage of previous lifetimes is released through forgiveness. I recommend using it repeatedly as you travel along your own path and become more and more ready to forgive.

This Higher Self Reiki technique can also be adapted for forgiving others for their acts against you in previous lifetimes. To do so, just say the following chant.

By the power of the golden light within
By the power of the sacred breath
I manifest this truth
I now will my Higher Self to send Forgiveness Reiki for the next hour
through my heart and my subconscious mind
to manifest forgiveness for all of the acts of harm others have caused me
in all of my lifetimes
I manifest this now
So be it!

(Blow three times.)

With both of these Higher Self techniques, it is hard to imagine that one invocation is going to manifest a lasting blanket of forgiveness that covers many lifetimes. But used repeatedly over time, these techniques can offer a deep release of lifetimes' worth of resentments. Use these techniques to release as much anger and resentment as possible, transforming those energies into forgiveness.

Free Yourself

The spiritual tools in this chapter teach you an effective and simple way to truly engage forgiveness. Many people talk about forgiveness but still harbor anger and resentment toward the person they say that they have forgiven. Forgiveness is a giant step toward spiritual awakening. And even if you are wading in the energy of Oneness and sending Reiki to yourself daily, if you are holding resentment or anger toward others—who are nothing more than mirror images of yourself—then you can never truly awaken to the Oneness that is your spiritual birthright. Take the time to use these tools for forgiving others and begin bathing your heart in the eternal spaciousness that Forgiveness Reiki provides during each session.

12

STEPPING BEYOND YOUR
KARMA WITH LOTUS REIKI

*A Lotus Reiki treatment has been sent to all who
read this chapter, to help in releasing any negative karmic debris from their energy system.*

Lotus Reiki works on releasing karmic debris from your energy system. This karmic debris is often what keeps us stuck in unwanted patterns of behavior. I was given this symbol by the spirit of Mikao Usui during the series of mystical awakenings I experienced during January 2007.

One aspect of spiritual awakening that some systems do not mention directly is the need to release those karmic energies that keep us trapped in illusion. Diane Stein mentions the importance of this in her book *Essential Energy Balancing* (see Bibliography, page 161), as do some other teachers of energy healing. But, in general, the idea of karmic release as part of spiritual awakening is too often overlooked. I believe, as one who has studied numerous energy healing systems, that karmic release is an essential ingredient in the process of spiritual awakening. You can have many blissful spiritual experiences, but if the energetic baggage that keeps you held in a place of illusion is not released, how can you ever truly awaken?

I mention this because it is important to distinguish between a spiritual high and spiritual awakening. Many people have glimpses of eternity, touching the Divine presence that is in all things. But once that glimpse becomes a memory, how do you still proceed toward awakening? I believe that the karmic energy that acts like grime on the window of the soul needs to be removed before you can always see the Oneness in all things, and live from that place of seeing. For it is when you begin to live from that place that you attain true spiritual awakening.

The Lotus Reiki Symbol

Lotus Reiki helps remove the karmic debris that is covering the window of the soul. The symbol for Lotus Reiki follows.

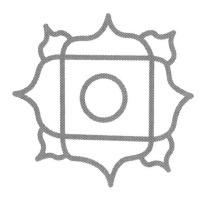

Lotus Reiki

You will soon be empowered with the ability to use this powerful line of Reiki light and will have the ability to use it in conjunction with the other empowerments you have received. Use it as often as possible to work on deep karmic release and clearing the karmic body.

Invoking Lotus Reiki

As with the other Reiki attunements sent through this book, it is important for you to meditate on what you wish to offer as an energy exchange to the Divine for receiving this sacred gift. Once you have decided upon an exchange, set aside a portion of your day or evening to take your cleansing sea salt bath. Then, dress appropriately and light a white candle to the Divine and Mikao Usui. Once you have done this and are ready to accept the transformational energy of Lotus Reiki into your life, say the following attunement chant:

Blessed are those who have brought us Reiki
Blessed are those who continue this sacred light
I and my Higher Self ask for the empowerment of Lotus Reiki
Blessings unto all
Blessings unto me

Allow this new light to embrace your entire being, knowing that you now have hardwired into your energetic system a spiritual tool that can unwind the threads of illusion, which have held you in a place of slumber, a sleep in which you forgot your truest nature. Lotus Reiki, perhaps as much as any tool in this book, has the power to unwind those threads, to release karmic debris from your system, and to allow you to see clearly once again that you are a whole and integral part of the One, the Divine.

As with the Forgiveness Reiki empowerment, this empowerment does not raise your overall vibration in the way that the first three Reiki empowerments do. Instead, it is allowing you more access to deeper lines of Reiki light that are designed for specific purposes. So I recommend using this new tool immediately to begin deepening your journey toward awakening.

Higher Self Lotus Reiki

Though Lotus Reiki can flow out of your hands if you are empowered with the Cho Ku Rei symbol, the most profound Lotus Reiki treatments occur in combination with the Higher Self. The easiest technique is to ask your Higher Self to send you a Lotus Reiki treatment for one hour. Do this before going to bed, as sleeping offers a perfect time for integration. Say the following chant before going to sleep:

By the power of the golden light within
By the power of the sacred breath
I manifest this truth
I now will my Higher Self to send a one-hour Lotus Reiki treatment
to my karmic body
I manifest this now
So be it!

(Blow three times.)

Know that you can adapt the preceding chant so that the focus is on a specific issue or you can use it for general karmic release: the choice is yours. Following is a chant for asking your Higher Self to send Lotus Reiki toward a specific karmic issue. All you need to do is choose a topic.

By the power of the golden light within
By the power of the sacred breath
I manifest this truth
I now will my Higher Self to send a one-hour Lotus Reiki treatment
to my karmic body
for the purpose of releasing karmic debris surrounding
the issue of [topic]
I manifest this now
So be it!

(Blow three times.)

Lotus Reiki is a powerful symbol, and it can have a profound effect on your entire energy system. On more than one occasion, I have seen a cloudy yellow light of karmic debris emerge from a person's spinal channel when using this symbol. I have also known some people (including myself) to try to move too quickly in using this symbol. Though it cannot do any harm, it can cause huge emotional releases that can be overwhelming. The symbol will cause change in your life, change for the better. But use it with patience and reverence. I recommend following any Lotus Reiki treatment with a Universal Reiki Integration Grid treatment. If you do a full hour of Lotus Reiki, then follow this with at least twenty minutes in the Universal Reiki Integration Grid.

13

ADVANCED REIKI TREATMENTS FOR SPIRITUAL AWAKENING

*A Divine energy treatment for releasing
the illusory veil of separation has been
sent to all who read this chapter.*

My path as a Reiki Master has been one of intense research. I have spent more time experimenting with the energy than I have in trying to create a private practice of teaching and offering individual healings. I have often thought of myself as a Reiki researcher, dedicated to the understanding of Reiki as an energy form and how it can be expanded and adapted into new forms for accelerating healing and awakening.

When I wrote *The Reiki Magic Guide to Self-Attunement*, one of the new techniques I discussed was the integration of the Higher Self into the Reiki process, which I referred to as Sahu Reiki. One technique that was born out of this form of Reiki is a Reiki Cord, which is like a little Reiki laser beam that can run between any two points in time and space for intense healing. To manifest a Reiki Cord, think of the two points in time and space between which you want the Reiki Cord to run. These are called Reiki Batteries, because they help add energy to the Reiki Cord, much as a battery adds energy to a flashlight.

Spinal Reiki Cord for Karmic Release

Reiki Cords can provide intense karmic release if you are using Lotus
Reiki and run them through the spine. This part of the body is where
most karmic debris is held. Reiki Cords can also offer intense healings
that help facilitate awakening when other symbols, such as Forgiveness
Reiki, are added into the process.

Following is an invocation you can use to run a Lotus Reiki Cord
through your spine. This healing can be intense and should be invoked
only when you know that you have a full day to yourself and can do
emotional processing afterward.

By the power of the golden light within
By the power of the sacred breath
I manifest this truth
I now will my Higher Self to empower my C-1 vertebra and my sacrum
as Third Degree Reiki Batteries
manifesting a Reiki Cord of Lotus Reiki between these two points
for the next half hour
I manifest this now
So be it!

(Blow three times.)

The Reiki Cord will manifest in your spine within a few seconds of the
final breath that you blow. Make sure that you follow this treatment with
a Universal Reiki Integration Grid treatment for at least ten minutes.

Higher Self Reiki Cord through Many Lifetimes

If you wish for a more powerful version of the same treatment, you can
ask your Higher Self to run the Lotus Reiki Cord through the time line
of your entire existence. Such treatments tend to be intense and are not
something I recommend unless you follow them with extended periods
of time in the Universal Reiki Integration Grid. Allow one minute in the
grid for every two minutes in which you have invoked the Reiki Cord.
To do this, use the invocation that follows:

By the power of the golden light within
By the power of the sacred breath
I manifest this truth
I now will my Higher Self to empower me in present time
and at that moment back in time when I first separated from the Divine,
as Reiki Batteries,
manifesting a Reiki Cord of Lotus Reiki between these two
Reiki Batteries for the next half hour
I manifest this now
So be it!

(Blow three times.)

The intensity of this treatment is something to be both cautious and excited about. Be cautious because it can bring up numerous unexpressed emotions, some of which are from previous lifetimes. And unless you properly integrate these emotions into your psyche by spending time in the Universal Reiki Integration Grid, the aftermath could be very difficult. Yet there is also great potential for deep karmic release from this treatment, which is why I include it in this book.

Experimentation

You now have numerous tools at your disposal for beginning to work on the karma that holds the veil of Maya in place within your own energy system. You can work on release of this karma at your own pace. For some, this work on the release of karma may require that they do many Forgiveness Reiki treatments. For others, it may require that they immerse themselves in the Universal Omega Reiki Grid or use Reiki Cords to run Lotus Reiki through the spine. For most, it will be an ongoing experiment using all of these tools. We all have things that we need to forgive. We need to forgive both ourselves and others. We all have karma from previous lives, or this life, that needs to be healed and released. And all of us can benefit from immersing ourselves, and the life situations we encounter, in the Reiki Grids. The cumulative effect of this work will be a shedding of fear, pain, sorrow, and the deeper karmic roots of these issues.

Combining Simultaneous Treatments

It is now time in your own evolution with Reiki to begin playing with how these tools best suit you. I recommend making a daily and weekly routine of using one or more of these tools. Sometimes it is best to combine them into simultaneous treatments. You can do this by layering and combining a number of these treatments to run simultaneously.

For example, have your Higher Self begin a treatment by sending Reiki to all of your lifetimes for releasing any karmic or spiritual blockages that have created separation consciousness in your energy system. Then layer that by putting the same issue into the Universal Reiki Healing Grid for the same amount of time. Over that, layer in a treatment of a Lotus Reiki Cord through your spine, or through many lifetimes, to work on any karmic issues related to the issue that you are working on.

Below is an example of how this would be done:

By the power of the golden light within
By the power of the sacred breath
I manifest this truth
I now will my Higher Self to send a thirty-minute Reiki treatment
to all of my bodies in all of my lifetimes
for release of karmic and spiritual blockages
I manifest this now
So be it!

(Blow three times.)

Then immediately add another invocation:

By the power of the golden light within
By the power of the sacred breath
I manifest this truth
I now will my Higher Self to immerse me
in the Universal Reiki Healing Grid
to work on release of karmic and spiritual blockages
for the next half hour
I manifest this now
So be it!

(Blow three times.)

Then, follow with this invocation:

By the power of the golden light within
By the power of the sacred breath
I manifest this truth
I now will my Higher Self to empower my C-1 vertebra
and my sacrum
as Reiki Batteries
manifesting a Reiki Cord of Lotus Reiki between these two points
for the next half hour
I manifest this now
So be it!

(Blow three times.)

After the thirty minutes is up and you feel the treatments come to an end, use the following invocation to immerse yourself in the Universal Reiki Integration Grid.

> *By the power of the golden light within*
> *By the power of the sacred breath*
> *I manifest this truth*
> *I now will my Higher Self to immerse me in the*
> *Universal Reiki Integration Grid*
> *to work on release of karmic and spiritual blockages*
> *for the next fifteen minutes*
> *I manifest this now*
> *So be it!*

(Blow three times.)

After the treatment has ended, stay well hydrated by drinking plenty of water for the next twenty-four hours. Get plenty of rest and sleep for continued integration. Also, know that the preceding option of layered treatments is just one possible scenario of options. Listen to your intuition—your own internal wisdom—when picking and choosing which tools to use, what life issues to work on, and the length of each treatment. Think of these Reiki tools as musical notes that you are learning to play so that you can be the pied piper leading your consciousness back into a place of Oneness with the Divine. You may develop your own kind of song, your own combination of these tools that works best for you. But as long as you keep moving forward, keep on forgiving, keep releasing the karmic barriers that keep your consciousness in a place of separation from the Divine, then you are headed in the right direction. For some, even a continual daily use of the blanket Reiki treatment across many lifetimes (shown in chapter 3) by itself is sufficient to begin to loosen enough karmic debris to allow real spiritual freedom in their lives. Whatever combination of these tools you decide to use, commit to a daily practice of a regular Reiki treatment and a weekly practice of a more in-depth, layered treatment. Your life will change in profound ways.

14

STEPPING INTO THE REIKI OF DIVINE CONSCIOUSNESS

A Reiki of Divine Consciousness energy treatment
has been sent to all who read this chapter.

During my experiences of mystical awakenings in 2007, one of the symbols shown to me was a Reiki symbol of Divine Consciousness. The importance of this symbol is that it can help loosen the veil of Maya, which keeps you locked in a place of separation from the Divine. When using this symbol, I do not send it to the emotional body, the physical body, or even the karmic body. I send it directly to the veil of Maya within my own energy system with the intention that it awaken whatever aspects of that veil are ready to be awakened at this point in time. The veil of Maya is created from Divine Consciousness that has fallen into a dream state, the dream of separation. By sending in more Divine Consciousness through this form of Reiki, you are helping the Divine Consciousness that is asleep—in the form of the veil—remember itself and awaken. Once reawakened, that Divine Consciousness no longer functions as a veil and no longer promotes the illusion of separation from the Divine.

Be warned that this is a slow and often methodical process. You will not awaken the veil overnight, nor is it likely that you will awaken it after a few weeks or even months. In fact, it is my own assumption that as long as we are in physical form, some aspect of this veil will always be in place. But, with effort and daily practice, you can begin to loosen the veil and at times even feel large portions of it slip away. As this veil begins to dissolve in certain areas, you begin to awaken to your natural state of Oneness with the Divine. Some spiritual teachers say that this veil can be broken down into various pieces, and that when certain aspects of the veil are released, it unleashes a spontaneous and permanent level of awakening. However, my focus has always been on the entire veil itself. This is not to say that I am right and these other teachers are wrong, just that from a place of Oneness, I see the veil of Maya as one veil with many different aspects. And I have found that surrendering into spiritual awakening as a process, rather than a goal, allows for some deep and fruitful work to continue on the self, even after significant portions of the veil of Maya have loosened and slipped away.

The Reiki of Divine Consciousness Symbol

To use Reiki of Divine Consciousness, it is important to visually bridge your consciousness into the symbol itself, though the actual techniques for using this symbol will be similar to the other Higher Self techniques mentioned in this book.

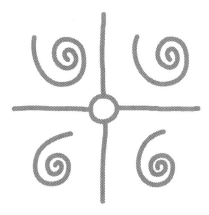

Reiki of Divine Consciousness

Invoking the Reiki of Divine Consciousness

As with Lotus Reiki and Forgiveness Reiki, you need to receive an empowerment in order to activate your ability to use this form of Reiki. Once empowered, you will have the ability to use the Reiki of Divine Consciousness. This line of Reiki light will deepen your journey of spiritual awakening by loosening the veil of Maya, which maintains your illusion that you are separate from the Divine.

As with the other Reiki empowerments sent through this book, it is important for you to meditate on what you wish to offer as an energy exchange to the Divine for receiving this sacred gift. After you decide upon an exchange, set aside a portion of your day or evening to take your cleansing sea salt bath. Then, dress appropriately and light a white candle to the Divine and Mikao Usui. When you are ready to accept the transformational energy of Reiki of Divine Consciousness into your life, say the following attunement chant:

> *Blessed are those who have brought us Reiki*
> *Blessed are those who continue this sacred light*
> *I and my Higher Self ask for the empowerment*
> *of Reiki of Divine Consciousness*
> *Blessings unto all*
> *Blessings unto me*

Allow this new light to fill your entire being, knowing that you now have hardwired into your energetic system a spiritual tool for awakening the veil of Maya, which maintains the illusion of separation from the Divine. As pieces of that veil awaken, you begin to see that you and the Divine are inseparable. Oneness is no longer something to strive for, but something that simply *is*.

Treating the Veil of Maya

As with the empowerments for Forgiveness Reiki and Lotus Reiki, I recommend diving right into this new Reiki form almost immediately after the empowerment. Begin by offering a Reiki of Divine Consciousness treatment directly into the veil of Maya:

By the power of the golden light within
By the power of the sacred breath
I manifest this truth
I now will my Higher Self to send a one-hour Reiki of Divine
Consciousness treatment
to the veil of Maya within my own energy system
I manifest this now
So be it!

(Blow three times.)

Let the treatment do the work of slowly reminding the veil that it is, in fact, nothing more than Divine Consciousness playing peekaboo with itself. The more you use this form of Reiki, the more you will slowly begin to remember your own true Divine nature.

15

CLIMBING INTO AWAKENING WITH REIKI HOLOGRAMS

A Reiki of Divine Consciousness energy treatment has been sent to all who read this chapter.

So far, all the work in this book has been focused on releasing the emotional and karmic obstacles to spiritual awakening. Though releasing the veil of Maya, and the karmic debris that holds that veil in place, is paramount to the journey of awakening, another important aspect of that same journey is unleashing the beauty and the power of cosmic imagination in our daily lives. This chapter and the ones that follow are not only about continuing to release obstacles to spiritual awakening, but also about gaining access to that childlike wonder and playfulness that often are the most powerful tools in this cosmic game of awakening.

Reawakening the Magical Child Within

As a child, you may have thought that you could create anything with your imagination. And on some level that is true. What we create with our imaginations as children affects how we see the world that we grow into. And, from a magical perspective, thoughts themselves are real. So for a child to imagine a unicorn means that at least a thought form of a unicorn came into existence with that thought. This does not mean that all mythological beings are human thought forms, nor does it mean that some children do not actually see fairies, elves, and other such beings. I believe that some children (but far fewer adults) actually do have interactions with such mythological beings. But regardless of your stance on this issue, the power of the human mind to create at an early and uninhibited age leads to a wonderful, playful way for a child to interact with the universe. And I believe that way of interacting, which is so precious and so often lost in adults, is also a path to God.

Jesus said, "Unless you change and become like little children, you will never get into the kingdom of heaven" (Matthew 18:3, International Standard Version). And though you could put various interpretations on what Jesus intended by this statement, for me it has always meant that we must embrace that childlike wonder and innocence that exist in all of us if we are truly to awaken to our own spiritual nature.

Reiki Holograms as Divine Play

Reiki Holograms not only provide new ways of healing, but also are a means of embracing your own sense of wonder and imagination in the process of healing and spiritual awakening. Once you become a master at using Reiki Holograms, you will have the ability to bring into this world in Reiki form anything your imagination wishes. And Reiki can do no harm. You will have a means of playing with the Divine.

Historically, most Reiki masters have seen Reiki as a form of light, something that exists in either wave or particle form. When someone sends Reiki, either through traditional methods or using Higher Self Reiki techniques, most often that Reiki is moving in wave or particle form, flowing through the body of the person receiving the Reiki treatment. You may have noticed that when you are receiving a Reiki treatment from another Reiki practitioner or from your Higher Self, Reiki seems to be *flowing* through you.

When I began experimenting with Reiki Cords, I noticed that there was less of a flow of Reiki and more of a constant *presence* of Reiki between the two Reiki Batteries holding the Reiki Cord in place. In other words, the Reiki did not seem to be flowing from one point to the next as much as it seemed to just *be there* between these points. As I experimented with this Reiki *presence*, I discovered that this presence can be shaped, molded, and infused with a specific purpose by the Higher Self.

What I came to realize was that just as scientists can use light to create a hologram, in a similar manner the Higher Self can mold and shape this Reiki presence into a holographic form to resemble anything in existence. I experimented and discovered that these Reiki Holograms can be infused with a goal of healing and spiritual awakening.

The beauty of Reiki Holograms is that they intensify both the healing and the awakening process and also open up the door for the universe to become a Divine playground. I have found that Reiki Holograms unleash a playful, innocent child in all who use them. And not only that: the power of a Reiki Hologram as a tool for healing and spiritual awakening is tremendous.

Reiki Holograms for Spiritual Awakening

I first began experimenting with this concept as a tool for physical healings, creating Reiki Holograms of diseased or injured areas of the body, intending that the Reiki Hologram be created to remind the tissue of its own perfection, to help bend it energetically back into a place of healing and light. For example, if someone had a neck injury, I would have my Higher Self manifest a Reiki Hologram of the person's neck, including all muscles, tendons, and other tissue, existing in a place of wholeness and perfection. Then, I would ask my Higher Self to merge that Reiki Hologram with the physical neck, which was injured. The Reiki Hologram would almost always create relief from the pain of the injury, and sometimes it would manifest a complete healing.

To use this technique for working toward spiritual awakening, you can create any number of Reiki Holograms, but one that might be best is to create a Reiki Hologram of your own karmic body, free from all clusters of karmic debris and free from any illusions of separation from the Divine. Reiki Holograms tend to fade out over time, so do not expect this to be a permanent healing. But what the healing will do is offer your karmic body a reminder of its own natural perfection, of a place that can be attained once enough karmic debris is released. To activate this, say the invocation that follows.

By the power of the golden light within
By the power of the sacred breath
I manifest this truth
I now will my Higher Self to manifest a Reiki Hologram
of my karmic body existing in its Divine perfection
free from all clusters of karmic debris and all illusions of separation
I merge this Reiki Hologram in now with my own karmic body
for as long as is for my highest good
I manifest this now
So be it!

(Blow three times.)

Notice how you feel after the invocation. You may be aware of a subtle but noticeable deepening of your sense of connection with all things.

Using Reiki Holograms

You can create Reiki Holograms to heal the body, expand consciousness, heal karma, and much more. There is only one limitation to their use: make sure that you are not invoking a Reiki Hologram on anyone else without their consent. One Reiki Hologram that I find particularly useful is one of the sarcophagus in the king's chamber of the Great Pyramid in Giza, Egypt. Having spent time alone lying in the sarcophagus in the Great Pyramid, I know that what transpires there has little to do with burial rites of the ancient Egyptian pharaohs and much to do with initi-ating people into their own cosmic alignment.

While lying in the sarcophagus, I had the sense that every molecule in my body was being cleansed and realigned for a higher purpose. Though a Reiki Hologram of that sarcophagus is not the same thing as actually being there, it will have a similar effect of cleansing and realigning your entire energy system. Before invoking such a holo-gram, make sure that you have someplace you can lie down to fully immerse yourself in this cosmic Reiki experience. As with many techniques in this book, I recommend doing this one while you are in your bed just before going to sleep. To activate this hologram, say the following invocation:

By the power of the golden light within
By the power of the sacred breath
I manifest this truth
I now will my Higher Self to manifest a Reiki Hologram
of the sarcophagus in the king's chamber of the Great Pyramid of Giza
around my own physical body
for as long as is for my highest good
I manifest this now
So be it!

(Blow three times.)

You will likely have incredible dreams using this hologram before sleep. And because the hologram is programmed to work only for as long as is for your highest good, it will fade out at the appropriate time. Usually, the process of sleep itself will provide integration when using this hologram. But if you use it while awake, then I recommend following it with time in the Universal Reiki Integration Grid, remaining in the grid for approximately twenty minutes for each hour that the hologram was in place.

Another wonderful way to use a Reiki Hologram is to create one of the time line of your entire existence since you first separated from the Divine. Infuse that hologram with the awareness of the bliss and serenity of your deepest connection with the Divine. Then, merge that hologram into that same time line of your existence. It is as if you are creating a second, perfect you, one that has never fallen from grace, and are merging that in along the time line of your many lives. It can have a powerful effect, helping you to remember your own true Divine nature. And because it is playful and fun, it allows you to do deep spiritual work and yet remain in that place of childlike wonder.

Create this hologram by using the following invocation.

By the power of the golden light within
By the power of the sacred breath
I manifest this truth
I now will my Higher Self to manifest a Reiki Hologram
of my entire existence, from that point where I first separated from
the Divine
through all of my lifetimes up to the present moment
and to infuse that Reiki Hologram with the bliss and serenity
of my deepest connection with the Divine
and to merge that Reiki Hologram in with the time line of my existence,
from that point where I first separated from the Divine
through all of my lifetimes up to the present moment
for [number] minutes
I manifest this now
So be it!

(Blow three times.)

Now, lie there and experience a deep sense of bliss and serenity, remembering the depth of your connection with the Divine. Allow this feeling to wash through you, merge into you, and echo in all of your thoughts and emotions. When this feeling has run long enough, release it. Or simply allow it to fade out once it has run for the specified amount of time. To release this hologram, state the following:

By the power of the golden light within
By the power of the sacred breath
I manifest this truth
I now will my Higher Self to release the Reiki Hologram
of my entire existence, from that point where I first separated from
the Divine through all of my lifetimes up to the present moment
I manifest this now
So be it!

(Blow three times.)

Experimentation with Reiki Holograms

A Reiki Hologram, like the other techniques in this book, can also be used simultaneously with more than one other Reiki Hologram or with other Reiki tools. In fact, using Reiki Cords, Reiki Grids, and Reiki Holograms together is one of the most empowering treatments you can offer yourself. The following is a series of simultaneous deep healings for spiritual awakening. You can make these deep healings part of your spiritual awakening practice once a week, as they are probably too intense for most people to use on a daily basis. Make sure that you are lying down when invoking a deep healing treatment, as it is very likely to take you into an altered, dreamlike state of consciousness.

By the power of the golden light within
By the power of the sacred breath
I manifest this truth
I now will my Higher Self to attune me in present time to be
a Reiki Battery
and attune me backward in time, at that moment when I first split
off from the Divine many lifetimes ago, to be a Reiki Battery
and to manifest a Lotus Reiki Cord and a Forgiveness Reiki Cord
between these two points in time through all of my bodies in all
of my lifetimes
I manifest this now for the next hour
So be it!

(Blow three times.)

Now, combine this healing with the Universal Reiki Healing Grid (or the Universal Omega Reiki Grid, if you want more intensity) by saying the following chant.

By the power of the golden light within
By the power of the sacred breath
I manifest this truth
I now will my Higher Self to put me in the
Universal Reiki Healing Grid
for the next hour
I manifest this now
So be it!

(Blow three times.)

Then, add a Reiki Hologram to further deepen the healing by saying the following:

By the power of the golden light within
By the power of the sacred breath
I manifest this truth
I now will my Higher Self to manifest a Reiki Hologram
of my karmic body existing in its Divine perfection,
free from clusters of karmic debris or illusions of separation
I merge this Reiki Hologram in now with my own karmic body
for the next hour
I manifest this now
So be it!

(Blow three times.)

Once the treatment comes to an end, put yourself into the Universal Reiki Integration Grid, so that you can fully integrate the healing, by saying the following:

By the power of the golden light within
By the power of the sacred breath
I manifest this truth
I now will my Higher Self to put me in the
Universal Reiki Integration Grid
for the next thirty minutes
I manifest this now
So be it!

(Blow three times.)

If, after the half hour in the Universal Reiki Integration Grid, you do not feel centered and balanced, invoke it again to deepen the level of integration until you do.

Please know that the preceding tools are entirely new to Reiki and that even most adept Reiki Masters have little knowledge of these new and transformational techniques. You can use these spiritual awakening tools for peeling away the karma that is the root of all separation from the Divine, as well as for becoming again a playful child on the Divine playground of life. You do not need a guru, a teacher, or any institution to facilitate this awakening.

What I have offered in this chapter can lead you to a place where you will begin to know your own true Divine nature, but you need to do your homework on your own. You must integrate Reiki Holograms—a form of Divine play—into your life, using them to remind you of your own true Divine nature. You can also use these techniques in conjunction with the techniques taught in the previous chapters of this book. Add these other techniques when it feels appropriate. The uses for Reiki Holograms are truly infinite. You can use them for physical healings as well as for deepening your journey to awakening. You can create Reiki Holograms of each organ in your body, infusing the energy of each to be in an awakened state. You can create Reiki Holograms of your own brain, and infuse your brain with specific states of awareness conducive to spiritual growth, such as the satori and nirvana states of awareness, mentioned in Buddhist texts on the path to enlightenment. The door is wide open, so wide that I cannot come close to mentioning more than a tiny fraction of the possibilities. Following is a template that you can use in your exploration of Reiki Holograms:

By the power of the golden light within
By the power of the sacred breath
I manifest this truth
I now will my Higher Self to manifest a Reiki Hologram
of [desired object]
and to infuse that Reiki Hologram with [desired energetic outcome]
and to merge that Reiki Hologram in with [where Reiki Hologram
should manifest]
for [number] minutes
I manifest this now
So be it!

(Blow three times.)

May your use of Reiki Holograms, and the awareness that their use will bring to you, shape your entire being deeper into alignment with that Divine presence that exists in everything, even the pages of this book.

16

LIFTING YOURSELF INTO HIGHER CONSCIOUSNESS WITH REIKI HALOS

*A Divine energy treatment to help loosen
the veil of Maya within you has been sent
to all who read this chapter.*

A halo is a luminous circle of light, either surrounding a heavenly body, such as the sun or moon, or, as portrayed in religious iconography, above the head of an enlightened being. When most people think of halos, they think of Christ, Buddha, angels, or saints with a band of white or golden light forming a circle several inches above the head. Many people acknowledge the halo as a symbol of being enlightened or spiritually pure. From an energetic standpoint, a halo is simply the radiance of an open and clear crown chakra (located at the top of the head), one that is so open that it creates a radiance that even those who do not normally see such things can tell is there. The halo itself is not the cause of spiritual awakening, but is rather a visual byproduct of an immensely open and clear crown chakra, which all enlightened beings have, even though not all people can see these halos.

Birth of the Reiki Halo

The idea of a Reiki Halo first came to me when I was offering a Reiki group healing to the staff of the Omega Institute. During the healing,

I heard a voice from one of my spirit guides tell me to invoke a halo made out of Reiki over everyone in the room. Then, as if I intuitively understood what this meant and the impact it would have on those receiving the healing, I asked my Higher Self to manifest a Reiki Halo over every person in the room. Immediately after invoking the Reiki Halos, I felt the consciousness within the room shift to a higher vibration. Since that day, I have used Reiki Halos both for personal use and group healings.

A Reiki Halo is simply an advanced form of Reiki Hologram. The purpose of a Reiki Halo is to raise your consciousness to a higher level by clearing the energy around the crown chakra and bringing your awareness to that area of your being. If you could see it, it would look like a halo made of Reiki, hovering several inches above your crown chakra. But because you are specifically naming this hologram a *Reiki Halo* (instead of simply a Reiki band of light above your head), it energetically also carries the infused energy of a highly spiritual state of awareness that is associated with a halo. In the same way, the Reiki Hologram of the sarcophagus in the king's chamber of the Great Pyramid is infused with an energy similar to that real-life object.

Using Reiki Halos

You can use Reiki Halos both as an adjunct layer in any of the layered Reiki treatments discussed so far, or as a separate Reiki treatment intended to clear the mind and bring your awareness up to a higher plane than your normal waking consciousness. The cumulative effect of using Reiki Halos is that it both creates a sense of spiritual bliss in the individual and also raises and focuses consciousness into the individual's higher chakras. The end result of cumulative use is a more spiritual outlook on life, combined with a clearer crown chakra and more serenity and peace in life.

The downside of a Reiki Halo is that, for some people, it might make them feel ungrounded. Therefore, I would use it only at appropriate times until you have gained such mastery over your own energy system that the Reiki Halo's effect will not keep you ungrounded or off balance. This mastery can be achieved by working with a variety of Reiki Holograms, creating ones for grounding that can balance out the Reiki Halo. Such a technique for grounding will be explained later in this chapter.

I recommend using Reiki Halos anytime you feel spiritually out of sorts or anytime you feel disconnected from the Divine. The deeply spiritual effect of Reiki Halos can usually remedy such problems almost immediately. To create a Reiki Halo, use the following invocation:

> *By the power of the golden light within*
> *By the power of the sacred breath*
> *I manifest this truth*
> *I now will my Higher Self to manifest a Reiki Halo*
> *three inches above my crown chakra*
> *I manifest this now*
> *So be it!*

(Blow three times.)

Allow the Reiki Halo to pull your awareness up toward your crown chakra while also cleansing this area of your energy system. Notice how the Reiki Halo makes you feel about yourself. It very likely will shift your thoughts to a lofty spiritual place. I usually allow a Reiki Halo to remain in place anywhere from ten to thirty minutes before releasing it. To release a Reiki Halo, repeat the following invocation:

> *By the power of the golden light within*
> *By the power of the sacred breath*
> *I manifest this truth*
> *I now will my Higher Self to release the Reiki Halo*
> *from above my crown chakra*
> *I manifest this now*
> *So be it!*

(Blow three times.)

Reiki Halos: Grounding and Integration

If after you first use the Reiki Halo invocation, you feel ungrounded, you can put yourself into the Universal Reiki Integration Grid immediately afterward to help ground your energy. And when invoking Reiki Halos in the future, you can add a Reiki Grounding Cord as a complementary treatment to keep you grounded.

To invoke a Reiki Grounding Cord, say the following:

By the power of the golden light within
By the power of the sacred breath
I manifest this truth
I now will my Higher Self to manifest a Reiki Grounding Cord
from my root chakra down to the center of the Earth
I manifest this now
So be it!

(Blow three times.)

Often, invoking the Reiki Halo has the effect of almost stretching an individual's consciousness upward into heaven. The Reiki Grounding Cord has the opposite effect, stretching your awareness into the earth. When the Halo and the Grounding Cord are used together, heaven and earth are connected through you, reaffirming your position as a spiritual being who exists in the physical realm. Use Reiki Halos daily to open your consciousness to a higher vibration, to lift your mind into the spiritual domain. As long as you do this with the mindfulness of remaining grounded and integrated, Reiki Halos will be a tool for stepping into higher consciousness each day and will accelerate your journey toward spiritual awakening.

17

STEPPING INTO
ENERGETIC ALIGNMENT
WITH REIKI PYRAMIDS

A Divine energy treatment to help loosen
the veil of Maya within you has been sent
to all who read this chapter.

Pyramids are three-dimensional architectural structures where the faces of the structure other than the base are triangular and converge to form a point at the top, called the apex. From an energetic standpoint, pyramids have the ability, through the perfection of their form, to amplify, align, and concentrate the energy that exists inside them. The most famous pyramids are those found in Egypt on the plateau of Giza, which some (such as the legendary Edgar Cayce) claim are remnants of a higher civilization that came to Egypt from Atlantis. In recent times, smaller pyramid structures have been used in New Age circles to assist with the energetic development of the individual, to deepen meditation, to heal, and to energize.

A Reiki Pyramid is a Reiki Hologram in the form of a pyramid. It is used to align and clear the energy of anything that is within a pyramid. Reiki Pyramids are not necessarily programmed to carry the energy of the Great Pyramid of Giza (or other great pyramids), though they can if that request is specifically made when invoking the Reiki Pyramid. Usually, I will create a generic Reiki Pyramid for aligning my energy system as a whole, and a more specific Reiki Pyramid, such as one that carries the energy of the Great Pyramid of Giza, for more intensive work. A generic Reiki Pyramid has the property of almost immediately bringing all my energy bodies into alignment and focus. And though this may not release karmic debris from my system, it does help me go through life with more focus and ease, which contributes to my ability to live a spiritually awakened life. If I wish a deep and mystical cleansing of my energy system, I will specifically invoke a Reiki Hologram of the Great Pyramid of Giza around my entire being. The effect of that hologram is more intense and something I do only when I have time to meditate and fully absorb the effects of the Reiki treatment.

How to Create a Reiki Pyramid

Creating a Reiki Pyramid simply involves asking your Higher Self to manifest it. It does not require any knowledge of the actual dimensions of the pyramid. You can manifest a Reiki Pyramid around not only physical objects, but also around situations, homes, offices, relationships (as long as all parties consent to it), or anything in need of an energetic alignment and tune-up. Think of the Reiki Pyramid as a cosmic mechanic.

Below is the Reiki Pyramid invocation:

By the power of the golden light within
By the power of the sacred breath
I manifest this truth
I now will my Higher Self to manifest a Reiki Pyramid
around my entire being
I manifest this now
So be it!

(Blow three times.)

Your Higher Self knows how large or small to make the pyramid; you do not need to specify its dimensions. In every instance, your Higher Self will create the pyramid so that you are at the center of it, receiving the greatest effect of its powers. An ideal amount of time in the pyramid may be anywhere from ten to thirty minutes, depending on the situation and how much of an energetic alignment and tune-up you want. To release the Reiki Pyramid after it has run for the desired period of time, say the following:

By the power of the golden light within
By the power of the sacred breath
I manifest this truth
I now will my Higher Self to release the Reiki Pyramid
I invoked around my entire being
I manifest this now
So be it!

(Blow three times.)

Once the Reiki Pyramid is invoked, you will likely begin to feel more focused, clear, and aligned energetically. When using this generic version of a Reiki Pyramid, it is usually not necessary to follow it with time in the Universal Reiki Integration Grid, though you can if you wish.

Using Reiki Pyramids

If you want to use a Reiki Pyramid for a particular situation, or around your home or office, you can do so by using the following template:

By the power of the golden light within
By the power of the sacred breath
I manifest this truth
I now will my Higher Self to create a Reiki Pyramid
around [person, object, or situation]
I manifest this now
So be it!

(Blow three times.)

I usually let a Reiki Pyramid stay in place when it is in use for an office, a home, or a situation. Often, it will fade out over time but can be invoked again and again as much as you desire for a long-term effect.

You can use the preceding template to help align aspects of your life, such as finances, career, or other situations, by naming that aspect in the blank part of the template.

For deeper spiritual work, you can invoke a Reiki Pyramid infused with the energy of the Great Pyramid of Giza in Egypt. Do so only when you have enough time for integration and processing afterward. The invocation for such work follows:

By the power of the golden light within
By the power of the sacred breath
I manifest this truth
I now will my Higher Self to manifest a Reiki Pyramid of
the Great Pyramid of Giza
around my entire being
I manifest this now
So be it!

(Blow three times.)

Once this form of Reiki Pyramid is invoked, you will begin to feel a deep alignment and cleansing of your energy system. You may want to stay in this Reiki Pyramid for thirty to ninety minutes, to allow its effects to permeate your entire being and all of your energetic bodies. This form of energy work will have long-term effects, helping you to shed energetic obstacles to spiritual growth and bringing you closer into alignment with your own Divine nature. Follow this invocation with time in the Universal Reiki Integration Grid. I recommend twenty minutes of time in the grid for each hour the Reiki Pyramid was in manifestation. Also, as with any of the more intensive energy treatments in this book, stay well hydrated by drinking plenty of water and get plenty of rest and sleep for continued integration.

18

WALKING UP THE STAIRWAY WITH GOD VIA REIKI HEALING EMANATION

A Divine energy treatment to help loosen
the veil of Maya within you has been sent
to all who read this chapter.

One of my favorite tools for using Reiki at the Higher Self level is a Reiki Healing Emanation Device. Healing emanation is based on a hands-on healing technique that I learned from Jason Schulman during his Three Pillars of Healing workshop at Omega Institute in 1995. The technique that Jason taught is simple yet profound. It speaks to the truth that the Divine exists within all of us, and within everything.

The technique I learned in that workshop has a simple premise: God will come into you if you only ask with a receptive and open heart. Keeping that premise in mind, if you lay your hands on another person for the purpose of healing him or her and then ask the Divine to enter you through your hands, the Divine essence that exists in that other person will rise up and enter your hands. Because that Divine essence emanates from the person upon whom the hands are laid, it calls forth a healing in that person as the Divine presence within him or her emanates forth. Unlike Reiki, this technique does not bring in Divine energy from the outside. Instead, it calls it forth from within the very person being healed. I so love this technique that I often use

it at the end of my Reiki sessions, even though the technique in itself
is not Reiki.

How Reiki Healing Emanation Evolved

As my path as a healer deepened, and I began using Higher Self Reiki
techniques, the possibility of using this healing emanation technique in the
form of a Reiki Hologram was revealed to me. I was shown that if I created
a Reiki Hologram of my own hands placed on myself or another individual
and then asked my Higher Self to program these Reiki Holograms with
the purpose of performing healing emanation, the Reiki Holograms would
indeed call forth that Divine presence in the person being treated. The result
would be a profound healing. I have used this technique both on myself
and other individuals and even in large groups. When using it in a group,
I simply ask my Higher Self to create numerous Reiki Holograms of my
hands on everyone in the room. There seems to be no limit to how many
people this can work on at any one time. At the moment I invoke this during a group treatment, the energy of the entire room shifts into a deeper
spiritual vibration, one that allows the presence of the Divine to emanate
through every body that is present and participating in the healing.

Reiki Healing Emanation can be a key to deepening your own relationship with the Divine. It surpasses that place of words and intellect
and allows for the presence of the Divine to actually be felt within the
body. Often people will mention seeing angels or other celestial beings
when this type of healing occurs.

How to Use Reiki Healing Emanation

To perform Reiki Healing Emanation on yourself, create a Reiki Hologram of your hands and ask your Higher Self to place this Reiki Hologram
on your body. Simultaneously, ask your Higher Self to program the Reiki
Hologram of your hands to perform a healing emanation. Generally, I
ask that my Higher Self place the Reiki Hologram of my hands on the
belly. If a more specific physical healing is necessary, then I will ask my
Higher Self to invoke the Hologram of my hands at the point of disease
or injury. But because this book is about spiritual awakening, and this
technique is an excellent way to deepen your connection with the Divine,
I will keep the focus of the placement of the Reiki Hologram of the hands

on the belly. But please know that you can place the Reiki Hologram of your hands on other areas, as the situation warrants.

I have also found that Reiki Healing Emanation does not take much time to lead me into a deep connection with the Divine. I tend to use this technique for only ten minutes, as the effect can be very deep and very profound even in that short amount of time. You can use it longer if you wish, but begin by simply doing a Reiki Healing Emanation treatment on yourself for ten minutes. It is best to do this when lying down, though it is possible to do this sitting in a chair. Try it first without using any other Reiki technique so that you can get a clear sense of what the treatment can do on its own. To perform this treatment on yourself, use the invocation that follows:

> *By the power of the golden light within*
> *By the power of the sacred breath*
> *I manifest this truth*
> *I now will my Higher Self to manifest a Reiki Hologram of my hands*
> *and to place it on the surface of my belly*
> *and to program this Reiki Hologram*
> *to perform a healing emanation on me for the next ten minutes*
> *I manifest this now*
> *So be it!*

(Blow three times.)

Be still and allow the Divine presence that exists within you, a presence that is endless and cannot be depleted, to arise through you into the Reiki Hologram of your hands, which lies on your belly. As this occurs, feel the deep presence of the Divine as it emanates forth through every cell of your being. To me, Reiki Healing Emanation feels like a light made of golden honey that rises up through every pore in my body and streams out into the space surrounding me. It is a wonderful merging of that latent Divine presence within you and your fully conscious self. Allow yourself to bask in this presence, to be held in this place of Divine love. And when the ten minutes comes to an end, breathe deeply into the sincere wisdom that has come to you while experiencing this treatment.

I do not generally recommend following this treatment with the Universal Reiki Integration Grid, though you may wish to invoke it if you feel emotionally overwhelmed by the experience. My reasoning is that any additional Reiki at this stage, even for integration, distances you from the direct experience you had of the Divine within yourself.

Later in this book, you will be shown how to use this treatment in combination with other Reiki techniques. But for now, at this stage of your spiritual journey, I recommend using it solo. In this way, you can engage more deeply with that Divine presence without confusing that presence with any other Reiki techniques or energies. Further on, I will show you how to use it in combination with other Reiki techniques in such a manner that the full impact of the treatment is entirely integrated into a larger layering process, one in which the true alchemy of Reiki is unveiled.

Drink plenty of water and get plenty of rest during the twenty-four hours following the treatment. Be kind to yourself. Be gentle. And allow the inner wisdom of the Divine to speak through you by calmly putting any insights you had during the treatment into action. Do not swim against the river, but flow with it. Hear and witness all that rises up inside you when you allow that Divine presence to be unleashed into this moment and into your life through the Reiki Healing Emanation practice.

19

STEPPING INTO THE MAGIC OF THE DIVINE WITH REIKI MAGICAL DEVICES

*A Divine energy treatment to help loosen
the veil of Maya within you has been sent
to all who read this chapter.*

My explorations as a healer and researcher of Divine energy have brought me to the conclusion that spiritual awakening does not have to be a stoic journey. On the contrary, it can be a joyful, energetic feast. There are so many pathways to the Divine that seeing this variety, and immersing your life in it, can unleash the multilayered truths of the Divine.

Reiki Magical Devices offer the opportunity to experience the truths of the Divine through multiple religious aspects. They also enhance your personal ability to gaze deeper into the looking glass of the soul and receive deep healings that open doorways to spiritual awakening. A Reiki Magical Device is simply a Reiki Hologram (usually of a power symbol from any spiritual tradition, or a specifically worded intent) that is imbued with a Divine purpose or active function. Power symbols can be the Christian cross, the Jewish Star of David, Buddhist mandalas, Pagan (or Christian) labyrinths, the Wiccan pentagram, Taoist magical symbols, and more.

Creating Reiki Magical Devices

To create a Reiki Magical Device, ask your Higher Self to manifest it, and then merge it into your body for as long as is for your highest good. The effect of each Reiki Magical Device will be different, depending on the symbol or intent you are using and its spiritual purpose. For example, when invoking a Reiki Magical Device of the Christian cross, I tend to feel a deep, loving energy of Christ focused in the region of my heart, then spinning outward, as if it has the effect of carrying this light far beyond me as an individual and out into the universe. The wonderful thing about a Reiki Magical Device is that it allows the symbol to affect you on a deep energetic level, bypassing many of the intellectual obstacles that can get in the way of direct communion with the Divine. The experience I have when invoking a Reiki Magical Device of the Christian cross is a perfect example in that intellectually I never would have assumed that one purpose of the cross might be to send Christ energy through the heart and out into the universe. And yet this is what I feel quite clearly when invoking this as a Reiki Magical Device. Experience this for yourself by saying the following invocation:

By the power of the golden light within
By the power of the sacred breath
I manifest this truth
I now will my Higher Self to manifest a Reiki Magical Device of the
Christian cross
and to merge this into my energy system
for as long as is for my highest good
I manifest this now
So be it!

(Blow three times.)

You may feel a strong presence of the light of Christ beaming through your heart out and into the universe after you invoke this. For me, this light is a form of Divine love moving from the Divine, through my heart, and out to all of existence. The impact of this allows my ego, my own sense of self-interest, to dissolve in favor of the higher wisdom of being compassionate to others, of loving others as I would wish to be loved. This feeling can be almost overwhelming for some and can be released if the intensity is too strong. To release this Reiki Magical Device, state the following:

By the power of the golden light within
By the power of the sacred breath
I manifest this truth
I now will my Higher Self to release the Reiki Magical Device of the Christian cross
merged into my energy system
I manifest this now
So be it!

(Blow three times.)

With the third breath you will feel the Reiki Magical Device begin to fade, but a residue of energy will remain for some time, due to the intensity of this particular device. Use this device to deepen your own understanding of Christ energy and how it pertains to your own spiritual awakening.

Infinite Variations

The preceding Reiki Magical Device is just one of the almost infinite options. There are as many such devices as there are sacred symbols of all the world's religions, plus more when you consider the other options, which follow later in this chapter. Use Reiki Magical Devices not only to perform healings, but also to deepen your awareness of the Divine. I recommend listening to your own intuition on what power symbols to invoke as Reiki Magical Devices. Let your soul speak to you through your intuition.

To invoke other Reiki Magical Devices, use the following template. You should probably begin with those symbols that have some resonance or familiarity to you so that you have some idea of what the effects might be. But know that often the effects will actually transcend any intellectual expectation. Use this technique for deepening your understanding of your relationship with the Divine by invoking whatever symbols

call to you. Following are some recommended ideas for Reiki Magical
Devices: the Merkaba flower of life; the Jewish Star of David; the Sacred
Heart; the Egyptian hieroglyph for Ab (the heart); the Buddhist dorje
or vajra; the crescent of Islam; yogic yantras; Wiccan symbols, such as
cauldrons, labyrinths, and the upright pentagram; Native American symbols and petroglyphs; and any other symbol of love, light, and connecting more deeply with the Divine. To invoke any of the preceding, use the
following invocation:

By the power of the golden light within
By the power of the sacred breath
I manifest this truth
I now will my Higher Self to manifest a Reiki Magical Device of
[symbol]
and to merge this into my energy system
for as long as is for my highest good
I manifest this now
So be it!

(Blow three times.)

Allow yourself to linger in the energy of whatever it is that you
invoked. Allow what you invoked to deepen your spiritual awareness on
an energetic level. If, at any point, the experience feels out of balance or
too intense, release it by stating the following:

By the power of the golden light within
By the power of the sacred breath
I manifest this truth
I now will my Higher Self to release the Reiki Magical Device of
[symbol]
that was merged into my energy system
I manifest this now
So be it!

(Blow three times.)

On your third breath, the device will be released and will fade from your energy system. You can use these devices as keys to unlock the deepest of spiritual truths through directly experiencing them as Reiki energetic forms. Using Reiki Magical Devices allows you to have direct experiences that can alter your awareness. You can begin to comprehend, internalize, and truly know what is sometimes only vaguely conveyed through the various interpretations of the world's most sacred spiritual texts. Use this technique to deepen your spiritual awareness through one spiritual path or through many spiritual paths.

The Tree of Life as a Reiki Magical Device
Another, more complex, Reiki Magical Device I often use is the Tree of Life from the Jewish mystical tradition of Kabbalah. The Tree of Life is an energetic map of all creation through a series of energy centers and energy pathways that can be related to the human body. Each energy center, called a Sephirah, emanates a particular vibration of the Divine. Traditionally, you can gain access to each of these Divine emanations through understanding and chanting the ancient Hebrew name of God that rules that particular Sephirah. Following is a diagram of the Tree of Life:

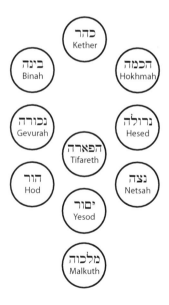

Tree of Life

When working with the Tree of Life, note that not only does Divine power emanate from each Sephirah, but that twenty-two energy pathways filled with Divine power and corresponding to each letter of the Hebrew alphabet also run among the ten Sephiroth (plural of *Sephirah*). A Reiki Magical Device of the Tree of Life radiates this Divine energy through your entire body. And bringing this energy into your body translates into shifts and changes in your life path that create a deeper relationship with the Divine. Because this Reiki Magical Device is so powerful, I recommend using it for only twenty minutes at a time. To invoke a Tree of Life Reiki Magical Device, speak the following invocation:

By the power of the golden light within
By the power of the sacred breath
I manifest this truth
I now will my Higher Self to manifest the Reiki Magical Device of the
Tree of Life,
creating a Reiki Hologram of each Sephirah,
infused with the Reiki energy of the Hebrew Divine name for that
particular Sephirah,
and to run Reiki Cords between the ten Sephiroth as energy pathways,
infusing each Reiki Cord with the Reiki of the
Hebrew letter most appropriate
for each particular pathway in the Tree of Life
and to merge this Reiki Magical Device into my energy system
for the next twenty minutes
I manifest this now
So be it!

(Blow three times.)

Allow yourself to absorb the treatment fully by lying down while this Reiki Magical Device is in use. Due to the strength of this treatment, you may decide to follow it with time in the Universal Reiki Integration Grid. When used repeatedly over time, this treatment can balance your compassion with your good judgment and bring you into a centered spiritual place where heaven and earth come together through the awakened Tree of Life that exists within you.

Reiki Shamanic Extractions

Another complex Reiki Magical Device is one I use for shamanic extractions. It relies less on sacred symbols and more on intent. A shamanic extraction is the act of a shaman pulling out negative energies, thought forms, or entities that have embedded themselves in your energy system and are disrupting your life and your spiritual growth. Once these energies, thought forms, or entities are removed, the body and energy system can return to wholeness.

To use a Reiki Magical Device for a shamanic extraction, first identify where the extraction is needed. This is usually an area where there is a consistent sense of the energy feeling blocked or where there is chronic aching, stiffness, or pain. Not all aching, stiffness, or pain is due to negative energies, thought forms, or entities, but sometimes they are the root cause. And in those cases, a shamanic extraction using a Reiki Magical Device can provide great relief. It can also reopen that part of the body and energy system to a greater degree of light and a more full expression of the body's original Divine intent as a temple for the soul. Invoking a Reiki Magical Device for the purpose of a shamanic extraction relies entirely on the wording, as no symbols are invoked in this process. The following page features a template for you to use, filling in the blanks where appropriate.

By the power of the golden light within
By the power of the sacred breath
I manifest this truth
I now will my Higher Self to manifest a Reiki Magical Device for
shamanic extraction,
to trap and cage any negative energies, negative thought forms, or
negative entities
in the area of my [organ or area of the body]
and to extend a Reiki Hologram handle from this device out beyond
the body surface,
which can be grabbed and held for pulling this Reiki Magical Device
and all negative energies, thought forms, or entities trapped within it
out of my body and my energy system entirely
I manifest this now
So be it!

(Blow three times.)

When you invoke this Reiki Magical Device, it will appear as a
cage of Reiki light that surrounds and traps whatever it is you intend
to extract. After manifesting this Reiki Magical Device, grab its handle
and pull the device out of the body, along with any negative energies,
thought forms, or entities caged within it. Make sure that you pull this
Reiki Magical Device clearly out of and far away from the body and
then offer the contents back to the Divine, to be either transformed or
redistributed to another location in the universe for the highest good of
all. To offer the contents back to the Divine, simply hold that as your
intention. You can call upon Kali, Jesus, the archangel Michael, or any
other heavenly being to take this energy and safely transform it or
relocate it.

Alternate Reiki Grids

The most common Reiki Magical Device is a Miniature Reiki Grid, which
is a much smaller version of the Universal Reiki Healing Grid. These
grids function in the same way that the Universal Reiki Healing Grid

does, but they are tiny and can be programmed to run over a specific individual or even specific areas of the body. The Higher Self creates holographic crystals of Reiki light, which surround the person or the area of the body to be worked on. Reiki Cords then link these holographic crystals of Reiki light to one another to form the grid. As complex as this process sounds, Reiki Grids are actually quite simple to invoke, as your Higher Self will know how to create them with only minimal instruction. Each Reiki Grid can be infused with specific energies, such as some of the preceding religious and spiritual symbols, or it can be infused with the energy of herbs, gemstones, other Reiki symbols, or any healing or spiritually empowering quality you wish.

One Reiki Grid that I find particularly soothing is the Reiki Rose Quartz Grid. This grid opens the heart center and holds it in a place of Divine love and compassion. Following is the invocation for the Reiki Rose Quartz Grid:

By the power of the golden light within
By the power of the sacred breath
I manifest this truth
I now will my Higher Self to manifest a Reiki Rose Quartz Grid
around my entire body and energy system
for [number] minutes
I manifest this now
So be it!

(Blow three times.)

The grid will fade after it has run for the amount of time that you specified. If you are using this grid in a general treatment for spiritual awakening, you might let it run for thirty minutes or longer. You can also invoke this grid when at work or when engaged in other activities. It will boost your love and compassion for yourself and others. In this case, let the grid run for only a few minutes; otherwise, the treatment might leave you feeling ungrounded.

Use the following template to experiment with Reiki Grids:

By the power of the golden light within
By the power of the sacred breath
I manifest this truth
I now will my Higher Self to manifest a Reiki [type] Grid
around my entire body and energy system
for [number] minutes
I manifest this now
So be it!

(Blow three times.)

The types of grids you can invoke may involve the energies of herbs, gemstones, crystals, or even songs, poems, or works of art. I often will invoke a Reiki Grid of a piece of classical music, such as Bach's *Air*, when I need a sense of calm and beauty in my day. This is where healing and spiritual growth merge into the realm of Divine play, and the magical child within reemerges and claims his or her rightful place on that Divine playground we call life.

20

ASCENDING INTO THE POWER OF RUNE REIKI

A Divine energy treatment to help loosen
the veil of Maya within you has been sent
to all who read this chapter.

Runes are a magical alphabet, much like Hebrew or Sanskrit, wherein the very letters and sounds of the alphabet are imbued with mystical power. Historically, Runes come from the Pagan traditions of northern Europe and are very much compatible with the journey of the Divine Warrior. Much of the energy that can be invoked through Runes has often been about hunting, winning, courage, and overcoming the obstacles of life. Traditionally, Runes have less often been associated with peace, communion, transcendence, or those virtues that can lead to spiritual awakening. And yet, for those who truly seek them, those qualities can be found in Runes.

The Place Where Opposites Meet

Because Runes have often been associated with the Divine Warrior and Reiki has always been associated with healing and inner peace, some might even feel that the traditions are mutually exclusive. Many among the Reiki community might say that any book on Reiki should have nothing to do with Runes. And, similarly, some traditional vitkis, those who practice invoking and using Runes, might feel that merging Reiki with Runes is an insult to a long, proud tradition of Runes that primarily honors the path of the Divine Warrior. Yet for me, there is a fail-safe method of bringing these two systems together that honors the best aspects of both traditions and also empowers individuals on their path of spiritual awakening.

I also believe that embedded in the mythology of northern European peoples is the very prediction of this merging. It is mentioned in tales about the Ragnorak (the end of the world), when the old gods and old ways will die out, to be replaced by a new spiritual order. As a student of Runes, I always found this tale to be a very sad one, as I hold a strong affinity with Odin, the Norse god who is said to have hung from the tree of Yggdrasil to gain the knowledge and wisdom of the Runes. I did not want to think that Odin, or any of the other deities I worked with in my study of Runes, could actually die.

However, in the summer of 2003, I was shown the deeper meaning of this myth. While creating a garden devoted to world peace with a shaman friend of mine, we were guided to place at its center a staff with several Runes written on it. This seemed odd to me, as I had always associated Runes with the Divine Warrior, not with peace. During the ceremony, when this garden was blessed for the purpose of peace, my shaman friend channeled a message from Odin, who clearly explained why we had been told to put the Rune staff in the very center of this peace garden. The message was that humanity had misunderstood the nature of the Divine Warrior and had thus abused Runes to create war instead of peace. The channeled message from Odin predicted that Runes would be transformed now to maintain peace instead of war and strife. My interpretation of this message is that the myth of the old gods and goddesses of the northern European pantheon dying is really about humanity awakening enough from our own spiritual ignorance to see Runes and the deities that rule them from a deeper, more awakened spiritual perspective. It is not that these deities will die, but that our own misinterpretations of them will die so that the true light of Runes and their deities can be revealed.

Practical Work for Spiritual Growth

Another reason for merging Runes with Reiki in this book is that Runes are very practical for the work of spiritual growth. Rune Reiki is very effective in helping to transform spiritual growth into real action in day-to-day living. Unlike the spiritual traditions that imply that we should hold ourselves apart from the physical world, Rune Reiki offers simple techniques to enhance our spiritual lives through how we live on a daily basis. Being a practical energy researcher, I have always favored honoring what works *through experimentation* instead of being guided by folklore, myths, or stories that could be misunderstood after being passed down through many generations.

Last, because Reiki works only for the highest good, these techniques cannot be abused or misused. Rune Reiki does not have the ability to do harm, because it is running Reiki energy from a Divine source and not running off the psychic energy of an individual's personal will or a group's collective magical will. This is essential to understand: Reiki can do no harm and is always for the highest good, and therefore the same is true for Rune Reiki.

The Elder Futhark

The Rune alphabet I work with is the oldest of all Rune alphabets and is referred to as the Elder Futhark. It consists of twenty-four Runes and is the alphabet from which most other Rune alphabets have evolved. When I teach classes on the Elder Futhark, I sometimes refer to it as an energetic table of elements because, with a good understanding of these Runes, it is possible to view anything in terms of the basic energetic components that these Runes represent.

Rune Reiki is the infusion of Rune energy into a Reiki Magical Device or Reiki Grid for the purpose of deepening toward the spiritually awakened state or taking that state out into the world through action. Any Rune in the Elder Futhark can be invoked by the Higher Self and used in a Reiki Magical Device or run as the energetic basis of a Reiki Grid. In either case, the person being treated with this form of Rune Reiki will experience an essential change.

Rune Reiki can awaken aspects of your own being, take you deeper into the knowledge of self, and also provide a stable groundwork for in-tegrating the more expansive techniques that have been explored in this book thus far. But to be able to use Rune Reiki effectively, it is essential to understand the basic energetic function of each of the twenty-four

Runes. Following are the Runes of the Elder Futhark, each with a brief explanation of its energetic function.

Fehu works to expand a sense of free-flowing
abundance and good luck.

Uruz is for healing, energizing, and strengthening;
it evokes the primal Divine masculine.

Thurisaz traditionally has some darker purposes,
but in Rune Reiki form, it is used to sharpen, focus,
and energize. It cannot be misused for curses in
its Rune Reiki form, as the Divine intelligence
within Reiki will not allow it.

Ansuz calls forth Divine inspiration and expanded
consciousness.

Raido helps in controlling and utilizing a deeper
sense of your own will and is especially good for
those who have abuse issues wherein their own
sense of will has been lost or damaged.

Cenaz revitalizes passion and provides knowledge
and wisdom about other planes of reality.

Gebo reconciles opposites, offering balance, blessings,
and integration.

Wunjo is often misinterpreted as "joy" but, in fact, is about coming into alignment with your deepest wishes, which then can create a joyful condition. If joy is lacking in your life, most likely you need to work on manifesting your true desires.

Hagalaz is traditionally about destruction and in the Rune Reiki form can be used to release negative life patterns. Meditating on this as a Rune Reiki Magical Device also brings you to a closer understanding of the transient nature of all things in that all in the world of form will eventually be destroyed and recycled into something new.

Nauthiz acts to constrict and limit and can be used to help ground an individual who is feeling overly expanded. For some, it can bring fears to the surface to be healed and can offer a person the ability to examine his or her own limitations.

Isa invokes the realm of ice and can slow things
down or even block an activity entirely. As with
Nauthiz, you can use it to gain an understanding
of your own limits. It is also very useful in
healing any kind of burn.

Jera (pronounced *yera*) invokes the positive
and gentle evolution of any situation over time.
It also has a gentle healing quality to it.

Eihwaz invokes courage, endurance, and motivation.

Perthro relates to hidden mysteries and the
womb and has the ability to awaken your
awareness of your psychic abilities.

Algiz invokes protection and is also a bridge
to higher realms of consciousness.

Sowilo calls forth the energy of the sun and can be
used for healing, energizing, and success.

Tiwaz invokes Divine order, leadership, and honor.

Berkana represents the nurturing aspect of the
Divine Feminine. It is wonderful for any aspect of
nurturing, such as renewal, rest, and regeneration,
and can also invoke protection for children.

Ehwaz works to create harmony and vibrations
of cooperation.

Mannaz activates the mind, intellect, and creative
thinking and is good for problem solving and
finding solutions.

Laguz deepens the connection with the dream
world and all things of a psychic nature.

Inguz is wonderful for integration and also activates
a connection with the fairy realm, thus inspiring play.

Othila, according to many, is the last Rune of the
alphabet, but I agree with author Freya Aswynn's
assertion that Dagaz is the final Rune. Othila invokes
the energy of community, the tribe, and connection
to what is important. It is also sacred to the god Odin.

Dagaz is the Rune of the Ragnorak, invoking
an energy of swift and extreme change. It is the
Rune that exists between realms, synthesizing
polarities, calling forth awakening, and taking
you deeper into the great mystery.

Rune Reiki Magical Devices and Rune Reiki Grids

To use Rune Reiki, invoke one or more of the preceding Runes as either
a Reiki Magical Device, which will call forth the presence of Rune Reiki
within your energy system, or as a Reiki Grid, which will allow Rune
Reiki to flow through your energy system. These two approaches differ
in how the Rune Reiki feels—a Reiki Magical Device is more of a presence and the Reiki Grid is more of a flow—but the general outcome will
be similar. You can also combine the two approaches for a deeper effect.
I recommend that you start by working through the entire Elder Futhark,
one Rune at a time, for a few minutes each. This way, you will gain an
energetic understanding of how each of them will affect you.

Following is a template for invoking a Rune Reiki Magical Device:

By the power of the golden light within
By the power of the sacred breath
I manifest this truth
I now will my Higher Self to manifest a Rune Reiki Magical Device
of the Rune [name]
and to merge this device into my entire body and energy system
for [number] minutes
I manifest this now
So be it!

(Blow three times.)

Notice the effect that this treatment has on your consciousness and your entire energy system. See if it changes your thoughts, your perceptions, and how you feel about yourself and the world around you. Should you need to release the treatment prior to its specified end time, use the following template:

By the power of the golden light within
By the power of the sacred breath
I manifest this truth
I now will my Higher Self to release the Rune Reiki Magical Device
of the Rune [name]
that was merged into my entire body and energy system
I manifest this now
So be it!

(Blow three times.)

After releasing the device, or after its specified period of time for running has ended, you may feel a residual Rune Reiki presence for a short period of time; this should fade within minutes. But know that even though the presence will fade, the effect that the device has on your energy system will be long lasting, especially if you continue to use the same Rune over time.

Some may prefer to use Runes with a Reiki Grid instead of a Reiki Magical Device, or to combine the two. Following are templates both for invoking and releasing Rune Reiki Grids.

Here is a template for invoking a Rune Reiki Grid:

By the power of the golden light within
By the power of the sacred breath
I manifest this truth
I now will my Higher Self to manifest a Reiki Grid
of the Rune [name]
around my entire body and energy system
for [number] minutes
I manifest this now
So be it!

(Blow three times.)

Here is a template for releasing a Rune Reiki Grid:

By the power of the golden light within
By the power of the sacred breath
I manifest this truth
I now will my Higher Self to release the Reiki Grid
of the Rune [name]
from around my entire body and energy system
I manifest this now
So be it!

(Blow three times.)

You may feel a residual Rune Reiki presence for a short period of time after releasing the Rune Reiki Grid. This presence should fade within minutes. But know that even though the presence will fade, the effect the grid has on your energy system will be long lasting, especially if you continue to use the same Rune over time.

Rune Reiki will not necessarily help you to release the veil of Maya. But what it will do is allow you to integrate your spiritual awakening into life through action. If the work of releasing karmic debris leaves you feeling vulnerable, you can invoke Berkana to nurture you and balance that release. Or if you need to feel lighter after the intensity of working with Lotus Reiki, invoke Rune Reiki in the form of Inguz to call forth your playful side. If the deep work of the previous chapters leaves your world feeling chaotic, which it might, you can balance that by invoking Tiwaz Rune Reiki to call order back into your life. The action-oriented aspect of Rune work, the palpable effect that it will have on your life, and the twenty-four energetic options you have with Rune Reiki make Runes an invaluable tool. Rune work will help you to maintain a balanced stride in life as you deepen your spiritual connection with the Divine.

21

DANCING ACROSS THE COSMIC RAINBOW WITH REIKI COLOR GRIDS

*A Divine energy treatment to help loosen
the veil of Maya within you has been sent
to all who read this chapter.*

Color affects consciousness. And using Reiki Color Grids can shift your consciousness toward a greater level of spiritual awakening. You can use Reiki Color Grids to work on numerous life issues as well as to more firmly establish and deepen the awareness of your connection with the Divine.

The Cosmic Rainbow

When working with color, I think about the rainbow. Rainbows are truly visual mandalas that depict our relationship with the Divine. Each of the seven colors of the rainbow corresponds directly to one of the seven chakras within our own bodies that govern our energetic well-being. And just as one side of the rainbow begins with red and leads eventually to violet, so, too, the chakras within our bodies begin with the red root chakra at the base of the torso and lead eventually to the violet crown chakra at the top of the head, which governs our relationship with the Divine. When you look at a rainbow, you are seeing the wonder of your own energetic system being revealed back to you as a beautiful and mysterious band of light.

The rainbow is a symbol of what it means to be both at one with the Source of all things as well as a separate individual. The colors that make up a rainbow come from the light of the sun, and yet each band of light has its own unique property and vibration. As the light of the sun, which represents spirit, enters into matter through droplets of water, the rainbow emerges and illuminates the sky with its beauty. Though each band of light within the rainbow has a unique identity, all those bands of light come from the same source, the sun. So, too, even though each person has a separate personality and a rich sense of self, all people come from the same light of the Divine, just as the colors of the rainbow all come from the light of the sun.

When working with Reiki colors, I use them to balance my own spiritual journey, and I usually start with the violet band of light.

Violet

Violet is the color you should use to deepen your communion with the Divine. This color relates directly to the crown chakra and in many esoteric practices is used to elicit wisdom and communion with the Divine. A Reiki Color Grid of the color violet can be used simply as a form of meditation, or it can be added to other Reiki practices and techniques you have learned in this book thus far. When using it simply as a meditation, let it run for a full half hour. If using it in harmony with other Reiki techniques as part of an advanced Reiki layering technique, then let your intuition be your guide as to how long the energy should run. Try invoking a Reiki Color Grid of the color violet as a meditation to feel how it raises your consciousness. After you have used it several times, you can then begin to experiment with how to adapt it to work in conjunction with other Reiki techniques.

Begin by using the following invocation:

By the power of the golden light within
By the power of the sacred breath
I manifest this truth
I now will my Higher Self to manifest a Reiki Color Grid
of the color violet
around my entire body and energy system
for thirty minutes
I manifest this now
So be it!

(Blow three times.)

Allow yourself the time and presence to fully appreciate the impact this treatment can have on you. Try it first when lying down at a time when you can devote your full attention to the effect the grid will have on your entire being. Again, know that you can use this form of the Reiki Color Grid to relax into your own innate wisdom and become more aware of your deep connection with the Divine. Let the grid do its work, but if you need to end it before the half hour is up, release it with the following invocation:

By the power of the golden light within
By the power of the sacred breath
I manifest this truth
I now will my Higher Self to release the Reiki Color Grid
of the color violet
from around my entire body and energy system
I manifest this now
So be it!

(Blow three times.)

Indigo

Once you feel comfortable with how the color violet works on you as a Reiki Color Grid, experiment with the color indigo. This color is associated with the third-eye energy center located between the eyebrows and is said to help open psychic abilities. Though an awakened third eye does not necessarily lead to spiritual awakening, it can enhance the journey and allow more information to come to you. To use a Reiki Color Grid to awaken your third eye, use the following invocation, again letting the energy run for a full half hour:

By the power of the golden light within
By the power of the sacred breath
I manifest this truth
I now will my Higher Self to manifest a Reiki Color Grid
of the color indigo
around my entire body and energy system
for thirty minutes
I manifest this now
So be it!

(Blow three times.)

Linger in this energy while it opens you more to your own innate wisdom and psychic ability. If you feel you need to release it before the half hour is up, use the following invocation:

By the power of the golden light within
By the power of the sacred breath
I manifest this truth
I now will my Higher Self to release the Reiki Color Grid
of the color indigo
from around my entire body and energy system
I manifest this now
So be it!

(Blow three times.)

Blue

The next color I recommend working with is blue. The color blue has two functions. Not only is it associated with the throat chakra, which rules self-expression, but blue also has a relaxing aspect to it that is good for helping you to sleep better or to surrender more deeply into a healing energy treatment. When I perform group Reiki treatments, I often use a Reiki Color Grid of the color blue over everyone in the room to help them go more deeply into a place of relaxation and surrender. As with the previous invocations of Reiki Color Grids, use this for a full half hour the first time you use it. This will help you fully absorb and know the impact the energy has on your entire being. Following is the recommended invocation:

By the power of the golden light within
By the power of the sacred breath
I manifest this truth
I now will my Higher Self to manifest a Reiki Color Grid
of the color blue
around my entire body and energy system
for thirty minutes
I manifest this now
So be it!

(Blow three times.)

This grid will make you relax so deeply that you may not want to release it! Let it run for thirty minutes and allow your entire being to drop into deep relaxation, which, in turn, can release any tension that might be blocking your throat chakra. If you need to end the treatment before the half hour is complete, use the following invocation:

By the power of the golden light within
By the power of the sacred breath
I manifest this truth
I now will my Higher Self to release the Reiki Color Grid
of the color blue
from around my entire body and energy system
I manifest this now
So be it!

(Blow three times.)

Green

The next color you should begin to work with is green. Green rules the heart chakra and is also said to be good for physical healing. It helps the body to release microbes and is a general tonic. As with the previous treatments, let this one run for a half hour. Following is the invocation for this grid:

By the power of the golden light within
By the power of the sacred breath
I manifest this truth
I now will my Higher Self to manifest a Reiki Color Grid
of the color green
around my entire body and energy system
for thirty minutes
I manifest this now
So be it!

(Blow three times.)

Allow this treatment to both open the heart chakra and heal the physical body. Remember that the journey to spiritual awakening includes taking care of your physical body and your emotional body. The color green assists in keeping both the physical body and the emotional body in good health. If for any reason you need to release the grid before the half hour is complete, use the invocation that follows.

By the power of the golden light within
By the power of the sacred breath
I manifest this truth
I now will my Higher Self to release the Reiki Color Grid
of the color green
from around my entire body and energy system
I manifest this now
So be it!

(Blow three times.)

Yellow

Yellow is the color associated with the chakra near the solar plexus, which relates to personal power. The student of esoteric practices may use yellow to elicit happiness, joy, and freedom from worry. If you feel depressed, disempowered, or sluggish, then using a Reiki Color Grid of the color yellow for a half-hour treatment can assist in healing those issues. To invoke such a grid, use the invocation that follows:

By the power of the golden light within
By the power of the sacred breath
I manifest this truth
I now will my Higher Self to manifest a Reiki Color Grid
of the color yellow
around my entire body and energy system
for thirty minutes
I manifest this now
So be it!

(Blow three times.)

You will feel as if the light of the sun is permeating your entire being when this grid is invoked. The Reiki vibration of the color yellow will emanate into all of your energy bodies and all of the cells of your physical body. It will soothe your troubles and cleanse your system energetically with its refreshing light. If you need to end it before the half hour is up, then use the invocation that follows:

By the power of the golden light within
By the power of the sacred breath
I manifest this truth
I now will my Higher Self to release the Reiki Color Grid
of the color yellow
from around my entire body and energy system
I manifest this now
So be it!

(Blow three times.)

Orange

The next color you should try working with is orange. Orange is the color related to the second chakra, located near the pelvic region. Esoteric literature says that orange works with the energy of attraction and success. A Reiki Color Grid using the color orange instills confidence. It can also be used to help attract what you want if you simultaneously add a visualization of yourself attaining what you wish while the grid is in effect. As with the previous grids, a thirty-minute treatment is recommended. Following is the invocation of this grid:

By the power of the golden light within
By the power of the sacred breath
I manifest this truth
I now will my Higher Self to manifest a Reiki Color Grid
of the color orange
around my entire body and energy system
for thirty minutes
I manifest this now
So be it!

(Blow three times.)

Some people may find that this grid actually brings their fears of success to the surface, which is a wonderful opportunity for greater healing and awakening to the truth of what those fears mean. If the treatment is overwhelming and you need to end it before the half hour is up, use the following invocation to release it:

By the power of the golden light within
By the power of the sacred breath
I manifest this truth
I now will my Higher Self to release the Reiki Color Grid
of the color orange
from around my entire body and energy system
I manifest this now
So be it!

(Blow three times.)

Red

The final color on the spectrum of the rainbow is red. It is associated with the primal animal aspects of your being. Red energizes, fights off infections, calls forth courage, and is the color most associated with direct action. If you need to get something done, red is the color you would invoke as a Reiki Color Grid to get you on your way. As with the previous grids, you can use this grid either layered with other Reiki techniques or as a solo half-hour energetic meditation treatment. The invocation for the half-hour treatment follows:

By the power of the golden light within
By the power of the sacred breath
I manifest this truth
I now will my Higher Self to manifest a Reiki Color Grid of the color red
around my entire body and energy system
for thirty minutes
I manifest this now
So be it!

(Blow three times.)

Feel the power of this color in Reiki form as it energizes your entire being. Know that it brings the cells of your body into a faster energetic vibration and helps the body fight infections when necessary. You can use this grid whenever you are ill or in need of a boost of energy and strength. If you need to release it early, use the following invocation:

By the power of the golden light within
By the power of the sacred breath
I manifest this truth
I now will my Higher Self to release the Reiki Color Grid
of the color red
from around my entire body and energy system
I manifest this now
So be it!

(Blow three times.)

Embracing the Rainbow Spectrum

As I mentioned earlier, the journey through the preceding colors is a journey through the chakras as well as through the spectrum of the colors of the rainbow. They are one and the same. One technique based on this concept that is particularly effective is to invoke the entire rainbow of colors at once. It has a psychedelic effect, grounding and expanding your consciousness simultaneously. You can experience this in Reiki form by using the following invocation of all the colors of the rainbow as a Reiki Color Grid. Immerse yourself in the awareness that behind each aspect of yourself, behind each fragmented part of your being, lies a greater whole, an indivisible whole that is part of the Divine. The invocation for this half-hour-long treatment follows.

By the power of the golden light within
By the power of the sacred breath
I manifest this truth
I now will my Higher Self to manifest a Reiki Rainbow Color Grid
around my entire body and energy system
for thirty minutes
I manifest this now
So be it!

(Blow three times.)

Your own sense of this treatment is better than any words I can use to describe it. Use this treatment to investigate your sense of identity within a paradigm of oneness, as paradoxical as that may seem. If you need to end the treatment before the half hour is up, use the following invocation:

By the power of the golden light within
By the power of the sacred breath
I manifest this truth
I now will my Higher Self to release the Reiki Rainbow Color Grid
from around my entire body and energy system
I manifest this now
So be it!

(Blow three times.)

Use Reiki Color Grids as part of your daily practice to maintain a steady balance on your spiritual journey. Staying grounded and integrated is essential whenever doing work that can expand your consciousness into a realm far beyond that of normal waking consciousness. You can balance or enhance your spiritual work by adding in the appropriate color in Reiki form.

Play with the Reiki Color Grids. Experiment. See what works for you. You are an artist engaged in the cosmic exploration of the soul. Enjoy the palette of colors in the form of Reiki Color Grids that you can use to shift your life and create a more balanced gestalt while on the path to spiritual awakening.

22

STEPPING INTO THE SACRED WITH REIKI PRAYERS AND REIKI MANTRAS

*A Divine energy treatment to help loosen
the veil of Maya within you has been sent
to all who read this chapter.*

My first experience with invoking a Reiki Prayer was in 1996, when a friend was visiting me at my apartment in San Francisco. The friend, who was a fellow Reiki Master, asked for my help in releasing an ongoing negative experience she was having with a misguided psychic, who was intentionally invading her energetic space. What I did not realize when I agreed to help clear my friend was how adept at manipulating energy this psychic really was. It seemed that every time I cleared away any negative energy from my friend, it would immediately reappear. At one point, after spending well over an hour trying to clear this situation energetically, I asked my Higher Self to attune two handmade ceramic plates to the Reiki of the Twenty-third Psalm. Though I had never attuned anyone or anything to the Reiki of a prayer before, I knew intuitively that this would help. I then asked my friend to stand on the plates so that the Reiki would flow up through her feet into her entire being. As soon as I did this, the situation changed and my friend became calmer. Within minutes after attuning the plates to the Reiki of the Twenty-third Psalm, we were finally able to clear my friend completely from the invasive energy of the misguided psychic. The potential and power of using Reiki Prayers has been known to me ever since.

How Reiki Prayers Work

A Reiki Prayer is that essential Divine spark, the core energy behind the words of the prayer, manifested as a Reiki Grid at the request of the Higher Self. I do not envision Reiki Prayers as a replacement for devotional worship or the act of praying, but I do know that they have a spiritual power that can accelerate the journey of spiritual awakening. Reiki Prayers can be from any religion, as they originate from the Divine spark within each prayer and are not limited by dogma or power issues. Though they use words to gain access to that Divine spark, they are a direct energetic "download" of the true essence of any prayer.

When working with Reiki Prayers, begin with those prayers with which you are familiar or feel some affinity. Eventually, you may want to include unfamiliar prayers, just to see how they shift your consciousness and to see if they open new avenues for you to know the presence of the Divine. Working energetically with a variety of prayers can give you an intuitive sense of what unfamiliar spiritual paths offer–their purpose and their appeal. It can lead you to appreciate religions that may seem alien as well as enhance your relationship with that spiritual path that is already familiar to you. For me, it has enhanced and helped heal my relationship with the Judeo-Christian traditions that once felt repressive.

Because your Higher Self has the wisdom and ability to gain access to the core energy of any prayer, you do not need to recite the prayer when doing the invocation to manifest the prayer in Reiki form. All you need is the name of the prayer that you wish to invoke.

The prayer can be a few minutes long or it can be quite long, depending on the need and intent of the person who is invoking it. To begin with, try working with prayers for five to ten minutes per day, just to gather a sense of how Reiki Prayers can affect your consciousness and shape your entire being into a deeper relationship with the Divine.

Following is how you would invoke the Lord's Prayer as a Reiki Prayer:

By the power of the golden light within
By the power of the sacred breath
I manifest this truth
I now will my Higher Self to manifest a Reiki Grid
of the Lord's Prayer
around my entire body and energy system
for the next ten minutes
I manifest this now
So be it!

(Blow three times.)

On your third breath, the Reiki Prayer will come into form as a Reiki Grid and fill you energetically with the Divine spark that is the core of that prayer. Allow yourself to be filled with this vibration of Divine light. If you need to repeat the prayer, or lengthen the time, do so by asking your Higher Self to do this and then offer three breaths of energy to your Higher Self to activate your request. If you need to release the Reiki Prayer before its specified time is up, chant the following:

By the power of the golden light within
By the power of the sacred breath
I manifest this truth
I now will my Higher Self to release the Reiki Grid
of the Lord's Prayer
from around my entire body and energy system
I manifest this now
So be it!

(Blow three times.)

You Higher Self will then release the Reiki Grid immediately after the third breath.

More Reiki Prayers

Prayers that I personally enjoy working with from the Judeo-Christian tradition are the Twenty-third Psalm, the Lord's Prayer, and the Shema (Deuteronomy 6:4–9). By working with these as Reiki Prayers, I have gained a deeper understanding of a tradition that I stepped away from many years ago. The Divine essence that shines through when invoking these prayers in Reiki form is much more palatable to me than the intellectual concepts. To experience prayer in Reiki form and bathe in Divine light, use the template that follows:

> *By the power of the golden light within*
> *By the power of the sacred breath*
> *I manifest this truth*
> *I now will my Higher Self to manifest a Reiki Grid*
> *of [name of prayer]*
> *around my entire body and energy system*
> *for the next ten minutes*
> *I manifest this now*
> *So be it!*

(Blow three times.)

Here are other empowering prayers that I have worked with as Reiki Prayers: Charge of the Goddess from the tradition of Wicca; the Iroquois Thanksgiving Address (an invocation that honors all beings and is never spoken the same way twice because it comes from the speaker's heart), and the Diamond Sutra of Buddhism. Each of these opens a new energetic avenue for relating with the Divine. Use what appeals to you when working with Reiki Prayers. The preceding prayers offer insight and wisdom for me, but they may or may not offer that same comfort to you. Experiment with other prayers, from whatever tradition calls to you personally, be it the Hail Mary of Catholicism, Islamic prayers to Allah, or other forms of prayer.

Reiki Mantras

Besides working with Reiki Prayers, it is also possible to work with Reiki Mantras. A mantra is a repetitious syllable or series of words that evoke empowered spiritual vibrations simply through speaking them. Mantras often contain one or more names of the Divine within them, such as Sanskrit names of various Hindu deities, Hebrew names of God, Buddhist names for enlightened beings, and Egyptian names for various realms of consciousness. It is possible to even create your own mantra, which is what most mystic poets actually do when creating an enchanting lyric that opens a door to the Divine. Such is the case with the devotional poems of the poet and Sufi mystic Rumi. The essential aspect of creating your own effective mantra is that the words transcend ego. The Divine is speaking to Itself through you. But before creating your own Reiki Mantras, first work with established mantras in Reiki form to again move deeper into your relationship with the Divine. Some easy mantras I have worked with that offer a great deal of wisdom and healing when invoked as Reiki Mantras are the following:

> **Sa Sekhem Sahu:** an ancient Egyptian mantra that translates as "the breath of life [sa], the power [sekhem], the fully realized human [sahu]."

> **Om Mani Padme Hum:** a Buddhist mantra that is dear to the Dali Lama and is said to energetically contain all the teachings of the Buddha. Generally, this mantra is used to evoke compassion.

> **Jehova Aloah Va Daath:** a Hebrew name of God that relates to the Sephirah Tiphareth within the Tree of Life and has associations with healing, devotion, and the archangel Raphael.

To invoke any of the preceding as a Reiki Mantra, use the template that follows.

By the power of the golden light within
By the power of the sacred breath
I manifest this truth
I now will my Higher Self to manifest a Reiki Grid of [name of mantra]
around my entire body and energy system
for the next ten minutes
I manifest this now
So be it!

(Blow three times.)

If you need to end the Reiki Mantra before its predetermined time, say the following chant for releasing it:

By the power of the golden light within
By the power of the sacred breath
I manifest this truth
I now will my Higher Self to release the Reiki Grid of [name of mantra]
from around my entire body and energy system
I manifest this now
So be it!

(Blow three times.)

Upon the third breath, the grid will be released by your Higher Self.

Relating to Aspects of Enlightened Consciousness

As you work with these Reiki Mantras, you will form relationships with various aspects of enlightened consciousness that will permeate your entire being energetically. The more you relate to these and expand your repertoire for experiencing the Divine, the deeper you will grow on your spiritual path. Eventually, you may wish to begin writing your own mantras, or devotional poems, to deepen your relationship with the Divine. One simple poem, which I was inspired to write many years ago and which I use as a mantra and invoke as a Reiki Mantra, is this:

Be loved by the Universe
By making the Universe
Your Beloved

You are welcome to try that poem as a Reiki Mantra, or write your own. By writing your own poem or mantra to connect you to the Divine, you are bridging your consciousness deeper into your connection with the Divine simply through the act of writing. Then, when you invoke it as a Reiki Mantra, you deepen that relationship energetically as well.

The ways of exploring your relationship with the Divine through Reiki Prayers and Reiki Mantras are endless, especially when you add your own devotional words into the mix. As a practice, this can strengthen the devotional aspect of your spiritual journey and help you step into a higher state. Use these techniques to explore new ways of experiencing the Divine, to grow familiar with spiritual traditions other than the ones you grew up with, and to water those spiritual roots that already exist.

23

ACCESSING THE LUMINOUS
REALM OF ANGELS THROUGH
REIKI PORTALS

*A Divine energy treatment to help loosen
the veil of Maya within you has been sent
to all who read this chapter.*

Angels are luminous beings charged to assist, and be spiritual
messengers for, the Divine. They can provide comfort, bestow
protection, offer wisdom, and give healing. In essence, they do the work
of the Divine in various ways. The angels most commonly known are
the archangels Michael, Gabriel, Raphael, and Uriel. However, there
are more archangels than just these four, such as Raziel, the angel of
wisdom. Interestingly, the angel that is said to be the most powerful and
closest to God is Metatron—yet Metatron is is not as well known as the
four commonly known angels listed above. To count the total number of
angels would be impossible. In fact, in Kabbalah, it is said that there is
an angel for every blade of grass. Some interpret this to mean that there
is actually an angel for everything that exists.

My many years of energetic and esoteric study have taught me that
there are numerous ways of connecting with these Divine messengers,
protectors, and healers. In some practices, there are sigils, or symbols,
that can be used to invoke a specific angel. During the sixteenth century,
John Dee, the astrologer for Queen Elizabeth I of England, channeled a

language he called Enochian, which supposedly allowed him to speak with the angelic realm; some still use that language to commune with heavenly beings. Others communicate quite easily with angels through prayer or simply the desire to communicate with them. In other New Age circles, contacting the angelic realm might involve a pendulum or a similar psychic tool. Personally, I have tried several of the preceding techniques but find that using a Reiki Portal is the most simple and effective way to gain access to the angelic realm.

A Reiki Tradition of Opening Portals

Opening portals is an established part of the Reiki tradition, though most people don't realize this. When sending Reiki, most practitioners right-fully use the Hon Sha Ze Sho Nen symbol to ensure that the Reiki arrives at its proper destination. But rarely in Reiki circles is it mentioned that this symbol actually functions as a portal. It's not a secret. It's just that many in the Reiki tradition have been taught to take things at face value. And because this symbol is not spoken of as a portal, most Reiki practitioners don't think of it as one. During my years of experimenting with Reiki, I have discovered that Hon Sha Ze Sho Nen can be used to gain access to the angelic realm—as well as other parts of the universe and other worlds—to bring energy from those realms into a Reiki treatment. And what better way to introduce the concept of Reiki Portals than to use Reiki Portals to connect with those heavenly beings who are among our greatest spiritual guides.

Opening the Portal

When opening a Reiki Portal to the angelic realm, make sure that you do so when you have time to meditate and be fully present. You may open either a general portal to the angelic realm or a portal to a specific angel. To begin with, I recommend opening a portal to the angelic realm and simply allowing their presence to be felt. I do this usually by opening the portal directly above my crown chakra so that the angelic energy flows directly into me. Use the invocation that follows.

By the power of the golden light within
By the power of the sacred breath
I manifest this truth
I now will my Higher Self to manifest a Reiki Portal six inches above
my crown chakra
by placing a Hon Sha Ze Sho Nen symbol there to gain
access to the angelic realm
I manifest this now
So be it!

(Blow three times.)

I have often used this technique in group healings and had the great joy of hearing that many people who were part of the healing either felt the presence of angels or actually saw them. Whatever your experience may be when you use this invocation, allow yourself time to appreciate that angelic presence, which so dearly wishes to connect with all of humanity. You may hear insights, feel a healing touch, or simply be aware of a soft and loving presence that permeates the room. When you feel that it is time to close the Reiki Portal, simply say the following invocation:

By the power of the golden light within
By the power of the sacred breath
I manifest this truth
I now will my Higher Self to close the Reiki Portal six inches above
my crown chakra
by releasing the Hon Sha Ze Sho Nen symbol placed there to gain
access to the angelic realm
I manifest this now
So be it!

(Blow three times.)

Connecting with Your Guardian Angel and Archangels

You can connect more deeply with your guardian angel using this technique: simply adapt the invocation to be more specific. Or use it to work with any of the archangels or other angelic beings that you feel drawn to connect with. Though there are too many powerful angels to list here, the ones I have worked with frequently are Raphael for healing, Michael for protection, Gabriel for guidance, and Raziel for revealing the mysteries of the Divine. You can work with any specific angel by using the template that follows:

> *By the power of the golden light within*
> *By the power of the sacred breath*
> *I manifest this truth*
> *I now will my Higher Self to manifest a Reiki Portal six inches above*
> *my crown chakra*
> *by placing a Hon Sha Ze Sho Nen symbol there to*
> *access the angel [name]*
> *I manifest this now*
> *So be it!*

(Blow three times.)

When working with angels in this way, you may even feel them move through the portal and enter the room. However you sense their presence, know that you can ask questions, receive healing, or simply bask in their love. By communing with these beings on a regular basis, you nurture an ongoing connection with them, which undeniably will result in spiritual growth. The exact outcome of your work with each angel may differ, but opening up to them and allowing them into your life and your energy field will deepen your spiritual journey to awakening. When you feel that you need to end your time with the angel, thank the angel and then close the portal in the same manner that you did when working with the entire angelic realm using the chant that follows.

By the power of the golden light within
By the power of the sacred breath
I manifest this truth
I now will my Higher Self to release the Reiki portal accessing
the angel [name]
I manifest this now
So be it!

(Blow three times.)

24

RAISING YOUR CONSCIOUSNESS WITH ELEMENTAL REIKI

*A Divine energy treatment to help loosen
the veil of Maya within you has been sent
to all who read this chapter.*

Western astrology, tarot, and other esoteric studies break the universe down into the four essential elements of earth, air, water, and fire. The element of earth oversees the physical realm, including issues of abundance and healing. The element of air pertains to issues of the mind and intellect and also rules things such as music and sound. Water is the element that rules dreams, the subconscious, and emotions. And fire is the element that represents will, passion, and creativity and also is the element of transformation. Elemental Reiki is used to invoke one or more of these elements in the form of either a Reiki Grid or Reiki Magical Device for the purpose of deepening the journey of awakening.

When I use Elemental Reiki, most often it is in combination with other Reiki techniques as part of a larger layered healing. The elemental work in itself will not release the veil of Maya, which holds the illusion of separation from the Divine in place. But what Elemental Reiki can do is work to maintain a balanced and integrated approach as part of a larger intensive Reiki treatment intended to shed the veil of Maya. The techniques that follow are part of the greater spiritual journey and help the soul to understand, at a deeper level, the nature of its own existence.

Element of Earth

The element of earth is the element I work with most. I use it to help with grounding and integration at the end of an intensive Reiki treatment. The effect it has is to bring your awareness back to your physical body. After invoking Reiki Cords through one or more lifetimes for intensive karmic release, or when using one of the other more intensive treatments mentioned in this book, I often end with ten or fifteen minutes of a Reiki Grid running the Reiki of the element of earth for integration. This can be used in addition to other Reiki techniques, such as the Universal Reiki Integration Grid, to deepen the level of integration. Should you wish to use this at the end of a session for integration, the template follows:

By the power of the golden light within
By the power of the sacred breath
I manifest this truth
I now will my Higher Self to manifest an Earth Reiki Grid
around my entire body and energy system
for the purpose of integration
for the next ten minutes
I manifest this now
So be it!

(Blow three times.)

Know that this elemental aspect of Reiki will help you focus again on your physical body and bring your mind back to the world of form. It is the perfect way to end a powerful and intensive session that might otherwise leave you feeling ungrounded.

Another use of the element of earth is to invoke it as a Reiki Magical Device in the body. Do this to help release stress or for a focused physical healing. Simply mention the intent as part of the invocation. For example, if you are using an Earth Reiki Magical Device for relaxation, say that in the invocation, which follows:

By the power of the golden light within
By the power of the sacred breath
I manifest this truth
I now will my Higher Self to manifest an Earth Reiki Magical Device
within my entire body and energy system
for the purpose of relaxing me on the physical level
I manifest this now
for as long as is for my highest good
So be it!

(Blow three times.)

A Reiki Magical Device with this intent will work quickly to assist the person in relaxing. Because the effect happens almost instantaneously, there is no need to put a time limit on the treatment. Other uses of this element as either a Reiki Grid or Reiki Magical Device include stabilizing, centering, enhancing self-esteem, and working on issues of abundance. Experiment with how this element complements your spiritual path by adapting either of the preceding templates to suit your purpose.

Element of Air

After working with the element of earth, begin working with the element of air. Because I am a Libra, which is an astrological air sign, I have a natural affinity for this element and love working with it. Usually, I will invoke it at the start of a treatment as a Reiki Magical Device with the intention of focusing my mind on Oneness with the Divine. Try this by using the invocation that follows.

By the power of the golden light within
By the power of the sacred breath
I manifest this truth
I now will my Higher Self to manifest an Air Reiki Magical Device
within my entire body and energy system
for the purpose of focusing my mind on Oneness with the Divine
I manifest this now
for as long as is for my highest good
So be it!

(Blow three times.)

Notice how this invocation almost instantly brings your mental focus into a place of Oneness with the Divine. You can adapt the preceding invocation to focus on other issues of the mind, such as clarity or alertness. You can even use it to solve a problem. Just use an appropriate phrase when mentioning the purpose of the Reiki Magical Device.

I use this element in the form of a Reiki Grid to cleanse my mental body, an energy body beyond the physical that holds our mental thought patterns, for about ten minutes each day. If you wish to include this technique on your own spiritual journey, use the invocation that follows:

By the power of the golden light within
By the power of the sacred breath
I manifest this truth
I now will my Higher Self to manifest an Air Reiki Grid
around my entire body and energy system
for the purpose of cleansing my mental body
for the next ten minutes
I manifest this now
So be it!

(Blow three times.)

Use both of the preceding invocations to play with using the element of air to shift your consciousness, raising it to higher levels.

Element of Water

Once you have gained an affinity for working with the element of air, explore working with the element of water. Remember, water rules the subconscious, dreams, and the emotional body (which exists beyond the physical and holds the deepest patterns of our emotional being). When I work with this element, I most often use it as a Reiki Grid to bring serenity to my entire being. Explore this yourself by using the following invocation:

By the power of the golden light within
By the power of the sacred breath
I manifest this truth
I now will my Higher Self to manifest a Water Reiki Grid
around my entire body and energy system
for the purpose of bringing emotional serenity to my entire being
for the next ten minutes
I manifest this now
So be it!

(Blow three times.)

Besides working with this element to find deep serenity, you can also use it as a Reiki Magical Device for assistance in remembering your dreams. If you use the following invocation every evening before going to sleep, it will help open the subconscious conduits to the dream world, which will result in healthier and more spiritually rewarding waking hours:

By the power of the golden light within
By the power of the sacred breath
I manifest this truth
I now will my Higher Self to manifest a Water Reiki Magical Device
within my entire body and energy system
for the purpose of opening the conduits to my subconscious and the
realm of dreams
I manifest this now for as long as is for my highest good
So be it!

(Blow three times.)

Using the preceding invocation over a period of time will allow you
to gain greater access to the power of your subconscious and the realm
of dreams. This technique can supplement your spiritual journey with the
amazing insights about life that often come to us when we dream. After
you have worked with the element of water, move ahead on your spiritual journey into working with the element of fire.

Element of Fire

Fire is the great transformer. It can both illuminate and destroy, bringing light or ashes to its cause. Fire also rules will, passion, and creativity.
Often, I use this element in the form of a Reiki Magical Device to bring
my will more into alignment with the Divine, which opens me deeper
into my journey of awakening. This technique can be done either as a
solo healing or as part of a layered Reiki treatment. Try it and feel the
wonderful quality of spiritual surrender that occurs when using this.
Following is the invocation for this form of Reiki Magical Device:

By the power of the golden light within
By the power of the sacred breath
I manifest this truth
I now will my Higher Self to manifest a Fire Reiki Magical Device
within my entire body and energy system
for the purpose of bringing my will into perfect alignment
with the Divine
I manifest this now
for as long as is for my highest good
So be it!

(Blow three times.)

Discover the effortless way in which spiritual surrender occurs when
using this technique. Not only does the Fire Reiki Magical Device affect
your will, but it also affects your entire body, which will often relax
from the effect of this technique. You can also adapt the preceding technique by changing the wording to create Reiki Magical Devices to work
on other intentions that relate to the element of fire, such as enhancing
your creativity or finding your true passion in life. Simply change the

purpose to indicate these desired outcomes and use the technique on a regular basis to see the results manifest in your life.

Besides using these wonderful forms of Reiki Magical Devices in my ongoing spiritual practice, I also invoke fire as a Reiki Grid to burn out anything negative within my energy system that is ready to be released. This, too, can be helpful in deepening into my true spiritual nature, as the fire element burns away obstacles on my spiritual path. Try this yourself by using the following invocation as either a solo treatment or as part of a more intense layered Reiki healing:

By the power of the golden light within
By the power of the sacred breath
I manifest this truth
I now will my Higher Self to manifest a Fire Reiki Grid
around my entire body and energy system
for the purpose of burning away all obstacles to my spiritual awakening
for the next thirty minutes
I manifest this now
So be it!

(Blow three times.)

This technique can release emotional and energetic obstacles that block your true devotion to your spiritual path. However, please note that a Reiki Grid of this type will not work on the veil of Maya. Only those Reiki energies geared for deep karmic release have the energetic capacity to work on the veil of Maya. Still, using this technique can supplement your growth on your spiritual path, allowing you the space and freedom to choose to continue engaging your spiritual work as best suits you.

Elemental Reiki can bring to your life the ability to influence layers of your being almost instantaneously. It can give you the opportunity to bring clarity to your mind and emotions in fast and effective ways, as well as simply ground yourself after an intensive Reiki healing. I work with this form of Reiki almost daily, and find it has made my life flow more smoothly and easily, and in ways that allow me to focus more deeply on my connection with the Divine.

25

CLIMBING WITH THE AVATARS USING REIKI TREE MAGIC

*A Divine energy treatment to help loosen
the veil of Maya within you has been sent
to all who read this chapter.*

Avatars are incarnations of the Divine, such as Christ and Buddha. These beings have no karma, no spiritual baggage that needs to be released when they incarnate into this realm. Their purpose is simply to spread Divine love and to work for the highest good. And though most people think of avatars incarnating only in human form, some believe that trees are avatars of the plant kingdom. If you have ever been among a grove of redwood trees, or in any forest that is pristine and untouched, you may understand why some people, including myself, think of trees as being some of the highest-level spiritual teachers.

Trees and Spirituality

Trees have a mystical presence that is enchanting and comforting and have been mentioned in spiritual literature for centuries. The Buddha is said to have become enlightened from sitting under the Bodhi tree. The Kabbalah expresses the Divine plan of all creation as a Tree of Life. Druids worshipped trees and worked with them often in their magical practice. In Nordic traditions, it is said that the god Odin hung from the tree of Yggdrasil to gain knowledge of the Runes. From a scientific standpoint, trees offer us the oxygen we breathe, keep soil from eroding, provide shelter to animals, and are essential to the ecological balance of the planet. No earthly being I am aware of provides such a multitude of positive functions, and thus it is easy for me to believe that trees are the avatars of the plant kingdom.

As avatars, and due to some energetic work that I did a few years ago, all trees now have the capacity to flow Reiki. My work to achieve this was performed in collaboration with the Deva (or Divine intelligence) that rules Reiki, the Deva that rules the tree kingdom, and my Higher Self. As part of this work, a mass Reiki attunement was sent to all trees on the planet that were willing to work with Reiki energy to promote planetary healing. When this attunement was given, it was intended to go only to those trees willing to work with Reiki energy. But shortly after the attunement, my guidance told me that because all trees are avatars, all the trees on the planet had accepted the Reiki attunement. Thus, it is now possible to work with any living tree as a Reiki healer.

Working with Trees

How I work with trees in this respect is to reverently ask my Higher Self to communicate with any and all trees in a general area, asking them to send Reiki to heal the land, heal community issues, or even add extra Reiki energy to an individual healing. If you want to work with just one tree, that is fine. But I encourage working with them as a group for a better and deeper effect. One way to begin doing this is to go to your favorite park or wooded area and have your Higher Self ask the trees in that area to send you Reiki for a short period of time. I never say this as a command, but always as a respectful request. Always approach the trees with reverence and as partners in healing. You can, if you wish, also send Reiki back to the trees, or bring offerings, such as crystals or other gifts, to show your gratitude. As long as you do it with reverence and care, trees are always willing partners, assisting your spiritual growth by sending you Reiki.

Following is an invocation for working with trees, which you can adapt as needed.

By the power of the golden light within
By the power of the sacred breath
I manifest this truth
I now will my Higher Self to contact all the trees in
[name of park or area]
and request that they send a Reiki treatment to
[person or issue receiving the Reiki treatment]
for the next [number] minutes
I manifest this now with gratitude to all these trees
So be it!

(Blow three times.)

Trees are amazing beings and working with them in this way will allow you to appreciate their beautiful presence even more. Not only does this type of work provide an unlimited number of Reiki assistants who can send you Reiki anytime, but it can also shift your consciousness away from human-centered paradigms of thinking that are the core of our ecological crisis. If for no reason other than shifting toward a more inclusive view of what is sentient and intelligent life, I recommend collaborating with trees as part of your daily Reiki practice for spiritual awakening.

26

STEPPING INTO ONENESS
THROUGH THE
ALCHEMY OF REIKI

A Divine energy treatment to help loosen
the veil of Maya within you has been sent
to all who read this chapter.

*A*lchemy is a word that implies transmutation. In the Middle Ages, an alchemist was one who was believed to have the ability to transmute common metals into gold through the use of mystical formulas. Today, many believe that the alchemists of the Middle Ages were less concerned with physical metals and more concerned with transmuting their own spiritual vibrations to a higher level. Thus I refer to the alchemy of Reiki as a series of layered Reiki treatments intended to transmute the sleeping consciousness that is the veil of Maya and awaken this consciousness to its own inherent Divine presence.

The Reiki layered technique that follows is an energetic formula intended to be used repeatedly until the veil of Maya awakens to its own inherent Divine presence. For a small few, it may happen the first time you use it. And for others, it may require a devoted practice that needs to be repeated for months or years to achieve the desired effect. The focus of this layered technique is to strip away karmic debris while also infusing the veil of Maya with so much Divine light that it cannot help but eventually awaken, much the same way you wake up when someone turns on the light in your bedroom. And just as some sleep more deeply than others, not everyone will spiritually awaken at the same pace when using this layered Reiki technique. Be patient. Know that each time you use this technique, you are stepping closer to union with the Divine.

An Alchemical Reiki Formula for Awakening

Most of the techniques that follow are based on ones you have used before. However, they are here specifically sequenced to assist karmic release and spiritual awakening at the deepest level—a real transformation that evokes the alchemy of times past. The fourth technique that follows is one not previously mentioned in this book. It is a request for energetic assistance from any other benevolent beings in the universe who want to assist in your spiritual awakening. True awakening is often as much a gift of Divine grace as anything we achieve by our own effort, so I have included this request for assistance in the following invocation sequence:

> *By the power of the golden light within*
> *By the power of the sacred breath*
> *I manifest this truth*
> *I now will my Higher Self*
> *to manifest a Reiki Portal six inches above my crown chakra*
> *to the archangel Raziel, who governs wisdom and awakening*
> *I manifest this now for the next half hour*
> *So be it!*

(Blow three times.)

By the power of the golden light within
By the power of the sacred breath
I manifest this truth
I now will my Higher Self
to manifest a Reiki Grid of Divine Consciousness
around the veil of Maya within me
for the next half hour
I manifest this now
So be it!

(Blow three times.)

By the power of the golden light within
By the power of the sacred breath
I manifest this truth
I now will my Higher Self
to attune all the vertebrae in my spine as Reiki Batteries
and run Lotus Reiki Cords between each and every vertebrae in my spine
for the next half hour
I manifest this now
So be it!

(Blow three times.)

By the power of the golden light within
By the power of the sacred breath
I manifest this truth
I now will my Higher Self
to call in any energetic assistance from other benevolent beings
in this universe
to awaken the veil of Maya within me
I manifest this now for the next half hour
So be it!

(Blow three times.)

Allow the preceding treatments to run for half an hour and then invoke the Universal Reiki Integration Grid, which follows:

By the power of the golden light within
By the power of the sacred breath
I manifest this truth
I now will my Higher Self to put me in the Universal Reiki
Integration Grid
for the next half hour
I manifest this now
So be it!

(Blow three times.)

Transmutation

Use the preceding layered technique to awaken and transmute the veil of Maya within you. This veil may take your repeated and devoted effort to awaken and transmute as it was created in that moment when you first split off from the Divine as an individual soul and it has been reinforced lifetime after lifetime. Know that it is very unlikely that just one treatment of this technique will be enough to entirely awaken the veil. But if you surrender into repeating this treatment on a regular basis, you will slowly peel away those layers of illusion that make you feel disconnected and separated from the Divine. After all, those layers are nothing more than Divine Consciousness that has fallen into a dream state of separation. Once awakened, the veil knows itself as Divine, and instead of acting as a barrier, it actually transmutes, becoming a bridge to a deeper state of awakened consciousness with the Divine.

27

THE GROUP REIKI TREATMENT

*A Divine energy treatment to help loosen
the veil of Maya within you has been sent
to all who read this chapter.*

Reiki is not intended for just the awakening of the individual. It is intended to be shared with friends and family and those who are part of our spiritual community. Offering Reiki group treatments is a way to create spiritual community, what the Buddhists call *sangha*. I have often seen many in new age circles who are primarily concerned with their own awakening and who shy away from extending the circle of light and awakening to others. If anything, this is contradictory to the idea of an awakened spiritual being, one who remembers always the Sanskrit adage of *Tat tvam asi*, or "That otherness is myself." When we begin to see that we are all of the same Divine being, compassion overflows into a desire to help awaken others on the spiritual path as well. Though it is not possible to take on the spiritual work of another, it is possible to open a door for anyone to step through and begin the journey to spiritual awakening.

A Group Healing in Seven Steps

The seven-step sequence that follows is recommended as an easy and simple way to share the work of this book with others and to create a sense of spiritual community without going so deep that it will overwhelm anyone. Though you should never coerce anyone into taking part in the Reiki group healing that follows, it is something that you can offer to energetically brighten your family, your circle of friends, and your community. This group healing will encourage them to work deeper on themselves, which, in turn, will assist in the awakening of humanity. Use the following sequence as a structure to share the gift of Reiki in a way that few have been able to until now:

1. Put the group into the Universal Reiki Healing Grid.
2. Invoke the Reiki Halo.
3. Invoke the Reiki Pyramid.
4. Invoke Forgiveness Reiki Cords through the heart (from present time back to birth). (Or run Reiki Cords through the organs and other areas of the body if they seem needed.)
5. Invoke Lotus Reiki Cords through the spine for karmic release.
6. Manifest a Reiki Hologram of each person in the group in a place of deep serenity and peace.

Allow the preceding functions to go on for twenty to thirty minutes; then release all the functions.

7. Put everyone into a Universal Reiki Integration Grid for fifteen to twenty minutes.

Afterward

After the treatment is complete, encourage everyone in the group to share their experiences. Also, remind them to drink plenty of water and get plenty of rest during the next forty-eight hours after the treatment. You may find that after a group treatment, many in the group are not very verbal, which is entirely natural. In such cases, you can encourage the conversation and sharing to occur at a later date.

28

REIKI ENERGY KOANS

A Divine energy treatment to help loosen
the veil of Maya within you has been sent
to all who read this chapter.

A koan is a word puzzle, a question that has no real answer within the normal context of time and space. Koans are used in the Zen tradition of Buddhism to assist students into a place of spontaneous enlightenment. Not all who are given a koan come into a place of spiritual awakening, but for some it is the trigger that causes that last bit of the veil of Maya to slip away. Perhaps the most famous Zen koan is, What is the sound of one hand clapping? There is no real answer, but pondering the question has led some students of Zen to a place of spiritual awakening.

What follows in the remainder of this chapter is a selection of what I call energy koans. These are mostly energy puzzles that evoke a questioning of reality as we know it. If taken to their deepest level, they can help open the door to your Divine self.

Energy Koan Number 1

Using the Higher Self Reiki techniques you learned earlier in this book, attune yourself in present time to be a Reiki Battery. Now, attune something outside yourself at a time in the past to be a Reiki Battery at the time you were born. Then ask that a Reiki Cord be manifested between these points in time and space. To simplify this, an example invocation follows.

By the power of the golden light within
By the power of the sacred breath
I manifest this truth
I now will my Higher Self
to attune me in present time as a Reiki Battery
and to attune Niagara Falls backward in time at the moment of my birth
as a Reiki Battery
and to manifest a Reiki Cord between these two points in time and space
I manifest this now
So be it!

(Blow three times.)

Traditionally, the answer to the koan is never given. But for this practice, because the koan itself is an energy puzzle and not a word puzzle, a few verbal hints can deepen the experience. If you work with this energy koan, you may notice a bending or shifting of time, a sense that you are experiencing in present time Niagara Falls as it was at the moment of your birth. For some, this energy koan experience is overwhelming, and if that is the case, then please ask your Higher Self to release it immediately. For others, this koan simply allows them to feel the fluidity of those laws that we take for granted as universal. Sensing this will allow your mind to deepen into the mystery of the Divine.

When you are ready to release this experience, say the following:

By the power of the golden light within
By the power of the sacred breath
I manifest this truth
I now will my Higher Self to release
the Reiki Batteries between me in present time
and Niagara Falls backward in time at the moment of my birth
and the Reiki Cord between these two points
I manifest this now
So be it!

(Blow three times.)

Energy Koan Number 2

Drawing again from the Higher Self Reiki techniques, create a Reiki Grid around your head that is attuned to the last digit of pi. Because the last digit of pi is only a concept and is, in fact, a number that is infinite, allow your mind to linger in this vibration as a form of Reiki coming to you through this Reiki Grid. Following is the invocation for doing this:

By the power of the golden light within
By the power of the sacred breath
I manifest this truth
I now will my Higher Self to manifest around my head
a Reiki Grid attuned to the Reiki of the last digit of pi
I manifest this now
So be it!

(Blow three times.)

To release this grid, use the following invocation:

By the power of the golden light within
By the power of the sacred breath
I manifest this truth
I now will my Higher Self to release from around my head
the Reiki Grid attuned to the Reiki of the last digit of pi
I manifest this now
So be it!

(Blow three times.)

This energy koan will allow your consciousness to linger in the energy of infinity. Again, some will feel overwhelmed by such an experience. If this happens to you, then release the grid immediately.

Energy Koan Number 3

Ask your Higher Self to manifest a Hon Sha Ze Sho Nen symbol in present time, linking you to yourself backward in time at the moment before you separated from the Divine. Allow your consciousness to linger in these two places simultaneously. Following is the invocation for doing this:

By the power of the golden light within
By the power of the sacred breath
I manifest this truth
I now will my Higher Self to manifest a Hon Sha Ze Sho Nen symbol
in present time,
linking me to myself backward in time at the moment before I
separated from the Divine
I manifest this now
So be it!

(Blow three times.)

For releasing this invocation, say the following:

By the power of the golden light within
By the power of the sacred breath
I manifest this truth
I now will my Higher Self to release the Hon Sha Ze Sho Nen symbol
that it manifested in present time,
linking me to myself backward in time at the moment before I
separated from the Divine
I manifest this now
So be it!

(Blow three times.)

Energy Koan Number 4

While lying down, ask your Higher Self to attune the atoms and molecules of your body to the Reiki of Yang and to attune the space between the atoms and molecules of your body to the Reiki of Yin. Allow your awareness to focus on these Reiki energies flowing into each other, which is what yin and yang do: they flow into each other and eventually each becomes the other. Following is the invocation for this:

By the power of the golden light within
By the power of the sacred breath
I manifest this truth
I now will my Higher Self
to attune all the atoms and molecules of my body
to the Reiki of Yang
and to attune all the space in between these atoms and molecules
to the Reiki of Yin
I manifest this now
So be it!

(Blow three times.)

To release this, say the following:

By the power of the golden light within
By the power of the sacred breath
I manifest this truth
I now will my Higher Self to release the attunement
of all the atoms and molecules of my body
to the Reiki of Yang
and to release the attunement
of all the space in between these atoms and molecules
to the Reiki of Yin
I manifest this now
So be it!

(Blow three times.)

Energy Koan Number 5

On an evening when there is a full moon, stand outside and ask the spirit of the moon if you can run a Reiki Cord between your own heart and the moon. If your intuition tells you that the answer is yes, then say the following invocation.

By the power of the golden light within
By the power of the sacred breath
I manifest this truth
I now will my Higher Self to attune the moon
as a Reiki Battery
and to attune my heart as a Reiki Battery
and to manifest a Reiki Cord between these two points
I manifest this now
So be it!

(Blow three times.)

Feel the cord of energy linking you to this celestial body. Allow your consciousness to bask in the fact that you are connected to this magical and ancient being. When you are ready, ask your Higher Self to release the Reiki Batteries and Reiki Cord, and thank the moon for the gift of this experience. Once you have successfully engaged this process with the moon, try it again with other celestial bodies, including the sun, other planets, stars, and even distant galaxies. Allow yourself to ponder then your direct relationship, which you have demonstrated energetically, with all of these celestial bodies.

Energy Koan Number 6

Ask your Higher Self to manifest a Reiki Hologram of your own brain, filled with the consciousness of the Cosmic Christ. Then, have your Higher Self merge this Reiki Hologram with your physical brain. Enjoy the effect of this Reiki Hologram on your own mind, knowing that eventually the Reiki Hologram will fade away. To invoke this hologram, use the following:

By the power of the golden light within
By the power of the sacred breath
I manifest this truth
I now will my Higher Self to manifest a Reiki Hologram of
my own brain
filled with the consciousness of the Cosmic Christ
and to merge this hologram with my own physical brain
for as long as is for the highest good
I manifest this now
So be it!

(Blow three times.)

Energy Koan Number 7

Ask your Higher Self to attune your name to be a Reiki Portal to the Divine. (A Reiki Portal on this level temporarily calls forth the innate Divine presence that exists within everything; in this case, the Divine will emanate from your name.) Now, say your own name again and again. As you say your name, notice the energy in your mouth, and how a Divine presence seems to emanate from among the letters you are mouthing. Think of the relationship between you and the Divine as you keep repeating your own name. Following is the invocation to do this:

By the power of the golden light within
By the power of the sacred breath
I manifest this truth
I now will my Higher Self to attune my name as a Reiki Portal
to the Divine
I manifest this now
So be it!

(Blow three times.)

The portal will eventually fade. But what will not fade is your memory of the Divine presence felt within your name as you chanted it.

Leaping Beyond

The preceding seven energy koans are simply suggestions of how you can leap beyond the normal framework of consciousness using advanced Reiki techniques. Though in and of themselves, the koans will not necessarily release the veil of Maya, they will offer you a wider perspective of your relationship with the Divine as well as demonstrate the malleable nature of time and space. This, in itself, helps expand and deepen your spiritual consciousness, allowing it to develop so that one day you will lose the veil of Maya.

EIGHTH-DIMENSIONAL REIKI

*A Divine energy treatment at the eighth
dimension for general healing has been
sent to all who read this chapter.*

Our daily consciousness exists in a four-dimensional awareness of the three dimensions of space plus the added dimension of time. But often, the root cause of an issue can be at higher levels, beyond these four dimensions. My own general rule of thumb is to assume that when it comes to the Divine, I should not try to put it in a box or set limitations upon it. So even though I often hear people talk about there being a set number of dimensions, I try not to assume that I know how many dimensions there are.

The Mystery of Dimensions

You might even say that dimensions are just another part of the illusion of separation and that to further fragment reality into more and more dimensions simply adds to the consciousness of separation. There are many ways to look at this from an intellectual perspective, and I do not pretend to have the ultimate answer on how many dimensions there actually are in this universe. But I do know that when it comes to energetic healing, it is possible to create an eighth-dimensional object.

What follows shortly is an empowerment to upgrade all of your Reiki abilities to work on an eighth-dimensional level. This empowerment will allow you to then flow any of these energies at the eighth-dimensional level simply by intending that this occur. Please note that most of the time you will not need to use this level of healing, that the Reiki techniques at the level you are already empowered to use are enough for most issues you will encounter on your journey of spiritual awakening. But sometimes, no matter how much energy you pour into an issue, nothing budges. In those instances, try using the eighth-dimensional empowerment for the energy work and then see if that creates more of a shift in the issue. Also, another reason for engaging eighth-dimensional energy work is simply to deepen your energy dance with the Divine, to come to a joyful recognition of how magical and wondrous creation truly is.

Eighth-Dimensional Reiki Empowerment

This empowerment will not be difficult to integrate if you have done the work in all the chapters leading up to this one. If you have not done this work, then do not ask for this empowerment. To do so would overwhelm your energetic system.

Before receiving this empowerment, which is the last empowerment in this book, you should once again meditate on an energy exchange with the Divine. Once you have come to a realization of what that exchange should be, and have made your commitment to the Divine to fulfill this energy exchange, then set aside a time and place that feels right for receiving this gift and for honoring the sacredness of this occasion. On the day that you are ready to receive the empowerment, take a sea salt bath to cleanse your aura. Once you have finished your bath, dress in a manner that fits the occasion and then light a white candle to the Divine and Mikao Usui. To receive the empowerment, say the following empowerment chant:

Blessed are those who have brought us Reiki
Blessed are those who continue this sacred light
I ask for the empowerment of Eighth-Dimensional Reiki
Blessings unto all
Blessings unto me

Allow your full being to linger in this experience. You may feel it in very subtle ways or not at all. The truth of this experience will be felt more when you are using this empowerment with respect to your own energetic practices. You now have the ability to flow all the energies taught in this book at the eighth-dimensional level.

There is no separate teaching for how to use the eighth-dimensional upgrade to your abilities. You will simply find it useful at times when you cannot get to an issue using other means. For example, if you are trying to strip away something at the karmic level, and Lotus Reiki is not going deep enough to get at the issue, try using an eighth-dimensional version of Lotus Reiki, simply by intending that it flow at the eighth-dimensional level.

Now that you have this empowerment, go back to any exercise from a previous chapter and repeat the exercise using an eighth-dimensional version of the energy called for in each exercise. This will become particularly interesting when you get to the energy koans, taking them (and yourself) to an even deeper level of awakening to the magic of the One.

30

AWAKENING TO THE DIVINE CHILD

*A Divine energy treatment for grounding
energetically into your human form has
been sent to all who read this chapter.*

During the writing of this book, I had a great lesson about embracing my own humanity. This lesson came to me through some profound personal healings. Perhaps the most profound involved allowing myself to go deeper into the grief of my own childhood. While in Bali, working on the last portion of the book, I became ill, feeling an odd energy in my right kidney that was combined with a fever and aching throughout my body. Turning to energy work for my own healing, I ran numerous Reiki Cords through the kidney, put myself into the Universal Reiki Healing Grid, and used every energy tool in my power to try to heal myself over several days.

Remembering Myself through Grief

The strange thing was that for months, a psychic friend of mine kept telling me that there was something in my kidney that needed healing. But every time I tuned in before getting ill—looking for bacteria, a virus, or some other ailment on the physical level—I could find nothing. The huge amount of light that was poured into the kidney during these days in Bali, however, unleashed a deeply buried childhood grief, a grief that felt like a small black rock that was sewed into the kidney itself.

156

For most of a week I was consumed by this deep grief, wondering what the lesson was for me. It is so often assumed that spiritual awakening takes us out of this place of human suffering. After all, for many people that seems to be the whole point, to bring an end to suffering. But what I learned while I was both in this immense grief and also going deeper into the energies of this book is that awakening is not at all about trying to escape the human experience. If anything, it is about learning how to be as human as you can be.

And who would I be if I were to turn off the pain of my own childhood by using the magic wand of spirituality? Would that be real spirituality?

I thought quite a bit about this while lying in bed, wondering why this lesson was happening as I was writing a book about awakening. And the conclusion I have come to is that the message was not just for me, but for all who read this book.

We Are Expressions of the Divine

The Jesuit mystic Pierre Teilhard de Chardin once said, "We are spiritual beings having a human experience." I do believe this, but would say instead that we are expressions of the Divine having a human experience. That we have fallen into the dream of separation was not a Divine error, but part of the Divine plan, a play in which the Divine could experience the myriad forms of consciousness we all embody.

When we use spirituality as a form of escape, as a way to avoid our pain, suffering, or passion for life, then we are misusing one of the greatest tools we have. The point of awakening is not to run away from life, to retreat from any wound, desire, or conflict. The point of awakening is to see the Divine in all of it. True, it does make life lighter and easier to flow through when you suddenly know that everything is Divine. However, having such an awareness does not subtract from the human experience: if anything, it adds to it.

Know Thyself

So why bother with all this spirituality if you are still going to suffer, still feel hurt and pain, and still experience all those other things that are a part of being human? Well, because the quest is, and always must be, simply to know thyself. And if you come to know yourself as part of a Divine being, then life does become lighter and more joyful but not to the point of erasing your own humanity. For remember, you have come into this body to learn about the human experience. Turn off all your emotions and senses, and that will never happen. But embrace them and see them as Divine, and underneath your tears there will still be a cherishing smile. The tears will not stop rolling, but they will taste sweeter against your lips once they have rolled down your cheek and into your mouth. It is not a spiritually embarrassing thing to cry, grieve, or feel anything that is part of the Divine experience of you.

Once during the workshop I mentioned previously with the noted energy healer Jason Schulman, he had us do a meditation on self-hate, where we simply sat and noticed those areas in our bodies and psyches where we held self-hatred. This experience led to another meditation wherein we noticed the anxiety our spirits had about being stuck in form. Eventually, all of these meditations of embracing *what is* lead to a state of what Jason calls *form preciousness*, where we as spiritual beings move through the self-hatred and the anxiety. And by moving through it, as opposed to avoiding it, we reach a liberating state where all that is in form has a new Divine flavor to it. The workshop lasted only a few days, but it has always stayed in my consciousness as a memory of how important it is not to use energy work or spirituality as a means to sidestep any emotion: not hate, not grief, not anger, nor any other human emotion. It is when we try to glide over these emotions or step around them that we short-circuit the truth. And short-circuiting the truth will never take you to the Divine.

It is this short-circuiting that often creates that stuffy atmosphere you find among some light workers who haven't done the real inner work. It is this imaginary heaven, or what I call shadow heaven, that some people seek that is entirely an illusion. And this shadow heaven unfortunately turns a lot of people off from anything spiritual, because they can see that something is not quite being said, that some very real emotions and agendas are being swept under the carpet.

The Divine Treasures of Being Human

In our grief, our anger, our fear, and our pain are some of the greatest treasures of being human, and of being Divine. The work of this book, and of awakening, is not about erasing those emotions or erasing your humanity. It is about embracing that humanity as an aspect of the Divine.

Take the tools of this book and use them in your life to create a better world and to create a better you. But do not assume that they will ever take you to a place where you are above sadness, anger, fear, or any other human emotion. You will likely live a more peaceful life due to this work, but that is not because you have amputated your humanity. That peace will come from peeling away the karmic issues that are the root cause of most suffering. It is not by hiding our tears that we become peaceful, nor by suppressing our anger, nor by being stoic when we are in pain. Peace comes when we awaken to the intricate connection we have with all things. Peace comes in knowing that even though we may be angry, in forgiving another we forgive ourselves. Peace does not come from imagining being peaceful when we are outraged, nor imagining we are enlightened when we are lonely. The only way to awaken, and the only way to God, is to embrace the truth. So whatever you feel when doing this work—be it joy, happiness, sorrow, grief, anger, fear, or any other emotion—simply be with it. Do not push it away or try to bury it. There is nothing shameful about being human. And when religions and spiritual paths awaken to this fact, then it will be easier for all of us to embrace the Divine, which exists in all things.

Do your spiritual work but also embrace your tears, embrace your desire, and embrace all that is you. And when you have done this deeply enough, and stripped enough layers of karmic debris from your system, you will meet that precious Divine Child that lives within all of us, a child who laughs when happy and cries when sad. To know Divinity at that level, in the innermost cracks of your human expression, in the places where you don't always look so good, is to find God.

Then you will want heaven on earth. You will want to be in love, because the lover, you know, is also a Divine being who gets grumpy at times, even as a Divine Child. And in the cracks and flaws of that relationship, you will discover an even deeper space of compassion and laughter and knowingness of your own Divine spirit.

Go then, out into the world with this *you that is changed*. And do not retreat from the world or hold onto the illusion that you can somehow hide from it forever. Go and take up the laughter you have always known lived inside your belly and allow it to explode loudly wherever you roam. Go into wild places and love and sing and be passionate with life, for you are an expression of the Divine, which has no need to hide its true form.

And if something slaps you hard in the face, allow yourself to weep. Or if a dear friend dies, allow yourself to grieve. Do not ever use the teachings in this book to hide from your humanity.

Being Divinely Human

We can now take this energy, this gift from heaven, and use it to raise ourselves up. We can attune our food to Reiki, offer Reiki to the land, and bring the tools of Reiki into every aspect of our lives. We can dance irreverently in this Divine play, with laughter and with hope. And yet always we should remember that if cut, we will bleed. And if inhuman to ourselves and the world, we will have failed in our Divine purpose of experiencing being human in this life.

Go then and be Divinely human. Be aware of the energies around you, above you, and within you, and use these energies to know the Divinity within life itself. Be as a Divine Child and feel everything that you were born to feel, and if you must suffer, then embrace that suffering as Divine. And if you feel the urge to laugh, then know that laughter as Divine. Be authentically you, for you are the Divine looking at me through these words as I write this book, and I would expect nothing less than that from You.

Bibliography

Andrews, Ted. *Simplified Magic: A Beginner's Guide to the New Age Qabala*. St Paul, MN: Llewellyn Publications, 1990.

Aswynn, Freya. *Leaves of Yggdrasil*. St Paul, MN: Llewellyn Publications, 1990.

Baginski, Bodo, and Shalila Sharamon. *Reiki Universal Life Energy*. Mendocino, CA: LifeRhythm Press, 1988.

Bevell, Brett. *The Reiki Magic Guide to Self-Attunement*. Berkeley, CA: Crossing Press, 2007.

Buckland, Raymond. *Practical Color Magic*. St Paul, MN: Llewellyn Publications, 1984.

Elson, Shulamit. *Kabbalah of Prayer: Sacred Sounds and the Soul's Journey*. Herndon, VA: Lindisfarne Books, 2004.

Masters, Robert. *The Goddess Sekhmet: Psycho-Spiritual Exercises of the Fifth Way*. Ashland, OR: White Cloud Press, 2002.

Stein, Diane. *Essential Energy Balancing*. Berkeley, CA: Crossing Press, 2000.

——. *Essential Reiki*. Berkeley, CA: Crossing Press, 1996.

Weinstein, Marion. *Positive Magic: Occult Self-Help*. Custer, WA: Phoenix Publishing, 1981.

Wright, Machaelle Small. *MAP: The Co-Creative White Brotherhood Medical Assistance Program*. Warrenton, VA: Perelandra, 1990.

Web Resources

For those interested in energy healing, go to www.brettbevell.com.

If you are looking for a good cause to offer time or money to as part of your Reiki exchange, explore the Cambodia AIDS Project at www.brahmavihara.cambodiaaidsproject.org.

Or you can help our environment by going to the Rainforest Action Network at www.ran.org.

Index

More from Brett Bevell

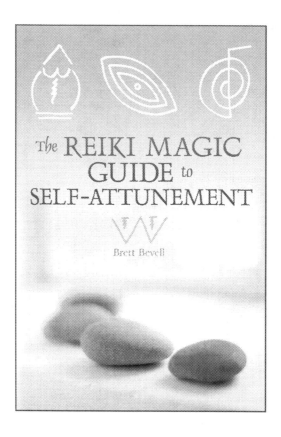

A revolutionary guide that extends the transformative powers of Reiki to all by presenting at-home rituals for self-attunement. Reiki Master Brett Bevell encourages creativity and experimentation, allowing you to personalize Reiki for everyday uses, including attuning stones, candles, the water in your bath, and more.

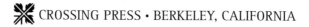

Printed in the United States
by Baker & Taylor Publisher Services